Journeys from Trust to Tragedy

By Norma Erickson

Dedication

"Tragedy is like a strong acid – it dissolves away all but the very gold of truth." **D. H. Lawrence**

The sole purpose of this book is to give a voice to all of the families around the world who found themselves dealing with mysterious new medical symptoms after HPV vaccine administration. Whether HPV vaccines caused or triggered these new symptoms or not is irrelevant.

The fact is the vast majority of them are suffering from real medical conditions. This needs to be acknowledged. Diagnostic criteria need to be established. Effective treatment protocols need to be developed. Anything less than this is a crime against humanity.

This book is dedicated to the brave souls who had the strength and courage to submit their personal experiences after HPV vaccine administration for publication and to the hundreds of thousands of others who have made similar Journeys from Trust to Tragedy.

In their honor, all proceeds from the sale of this book will be donated to SaneVax Inc., and AHVID.

Contents

Acknowledgements

This book would not exist without the invaluable assistance the author received from Freda Birrell. She worked tirelessly to gather stories from families who have been forced to deal with the serious new medical conditions their children experienced after the administration of HPV vaccines. Freda took the time to personally examine every single page to make sure the author did not include any typographical errors. She was an invaluable liaison between the author and families as the stories were passed back and forth throughout the editing process. Most remarkable of all, she accomplished all of this while keeping up with her responsibilities as Chair of AHVID (UK association of HPV vaccine-injured daughters) and doing a phenomenal job as Public Relations Director and Secretary of SaneVax.

On a similar note, without the courage and strength of those families who submitted stories, this book would not exist. Society owes them a huge debt of gratitude for having the fortitude to open their lives to public scrutiny in order to try and prevent others from making the same journey they have been forced to travel. We often tend to forget that it is not just the person with new medical symptoms who is suffering. It is their entire family, their circle of friends, their community, and indeed society as a whole. The world will never know how much these injured individuals would have contributed to humanity had they not been assaulted with a multitude of debilitating medical conditions during their youth. Who knows what would have happened if medical professionals had listened to them and tried to find out what was causing their new health problems. Who knows what would have happened if doctors had looked for ways to cure them instead of taking the 'it can't be the vaccine' stance.

We must also recognize the contribution made by the manufacturers of HPV vaccines, the health authorities who approved their use and the government authorities and others who promoted them. Without all of these entities pushing so hard for vaccine uptake while ignoring the cries of those who were injured, these families would have never have had to resort to networking with each other for help. If medical professionals had simply listened and tried to discover causes and effective treatments, these families would have never turned to outside sources for answers. They would not have needed to become the international voice for change they have been forced to become. They would not have needed to become a force strong enough to create a world where this type of disaster will not be tolerated without first having been injected and neglected.

Preface

In 1971, the United States President Richard M. Nixon officially declared war on cancer in response to public demand for cures. At the time, cancer was the second leading cause of death in the United States, right behind heart attacks. President Nixon promised to ask for one hundred million dollars' worth of funding to begin the battle. [1]

The National Cancer Act passed through Congress with bipartisan support and was signed into law on December 23, 1971. Congress set aside an unprecedented 1.6 billion dollars in federal funding for cancer research.[2] Almost immediately, various scientific research entities began to dive into the newly established pool of funds.

During the ensuing years the National Cancer Institute spent 90 billion dollars on cancer research and treatments. This does not take into account the nearly 2.2 billion dollars invested by the 260 non-profit organizations in the United States that are dedicated to fighting cancer.

Needless to say, competition for these funds became intense quickly.

In 1983-84, Professor Harald zur Hausen discovered HPV 16 and 18 DNA in cervical cancer cell lines.

There was no concrete evidence HPV 16/18 were causal agents of said cancer cell lines, simply an association between the two existed. [3,4]

As stated in the *NIH Registry,* "NIH's Office of Technology Transfer (OTT) was created by NIH in 1989 to evaluate, protect, license and

---

[1] US National Cancer Institute; Milestone (1971)

[2] Russell, Sabin; Nixon's War on Cancer: Why it mattered; Sept 2016; Fred Hutch News Service; accessed March 2019

[3] Durst M, Gissmann L, Ikenberg H, zur Hausen H: A papillomavirus DNA from a cervical carcinoma and its prevalence in cancer biopsy samples from different geographic regions. Proc Natl Acad Sci USA 1983; 80:3812-3815.

[4] Boshart M, Gissmann L, Ikenberg H, Kleinheinz A, Scheurlen W, zur Hausen H: A new type of papillomavirus DNA, its presence in genital cancer biopsies and in cell lines derived from cervical cancer. EMBO J 1984, 3:1151-1157.

manage both NIH and FDA discoveries, inventions and other intellectual property."[5]

The OTT turned out to be a timely creation, because from July 1991 through August 2007, there were multiple patents filed along with subsequent court battles to determine who actually owned the patent rights to production methods for HPV vaccines.[6]

In spite of the fact that patent right ownership would not be determined for another year, the first HPV vaccine, Gardasil was granted FDA approval on June 8, 2006.

It is interesting to note that at the time of approval, the HHS definition of 'vaccine' was, *"a product of a weakened or killed microorganism (bacteria or virus) given for the prevention or treatment of an infectious disease."*[7]

Everyone knows infection is not synonymous with an infectious disease. You cannot 'catch' cancer from someone else. Therefore, it is not an infectious disease. By the HHS definition, any injection administered to protect against cancer of any type did not fit the definition of 'vaccine'.

When the SaneVax team pointed out this problem, the HHS decided to change the definition of 'vaccine' to *"A product that produces immunity therefore protecting the body from the disease. Vaccines are administered through needle injections, by mouth and by aerosol."*

Evidently, the officials at HHS determined that it was more expedient to protect their patent rights than to investigate the possibility of consumer fraud. Could this have anything to do with the fact that the National Institutes of Health receive an undisclosed amount of royalties[8] from the sale of HPV vaccines because they own patent rights?

If the original definition of 'vaccine' were adhered to, manufacturers of this medical intervention could be held responsible for the quality and safety of their products.

---

[5] NIH Record (02/23/2007); *Bridging the Licensing Gap,* by Sarah Schmelling

[6] Erickson, Norma; Creating an HPV Industry; April 2011; accessed March 2019;

[7] Erickson, Norma; How far will tax-payer sponsored health agencies go to protect HPV vaccines?; Oct 2011; accessed March 2019

[8] Nisbet, Miriam; Response to FOI request no. 2011-0059; National Archives and Records Administration (OGIS); accessed March 2019

As 'vaccines' they fall under the purview of the National Vaccine Injury Compensation Program which was created after the National Childhood Vaccine Injury Act of 1986.[9] This granted vaccine stakeholders virtual immunity from prosecution for vaccine injuries. All claims for vaccine injury would have to be filed under the NVICP before the family involved could even consider filing a claim in a traditional court.

According to the World Health Organization, between 2006 and 2017, 270 million doses of HPV vaccines were distributed[10] around the world. If one assumes that only half of those doses have been administered, according to the clinical trial data Merck submitted to the FDA prior to Gardasil approval, there should be approximately 3 million young people around the world who experienced serious new medical conditions potentially indicative of an autoimmune disorder.

If that is true, the families in this book are barely the tip of the iceberg. It may take decades to uncover the amount of destruction left in the wake of HPV vaccination programs.

Potentially 3 million families whose lives have been changed forever: Is this acceptable, collateral damage when conducting a 'war on cancer'?

---

[9]The College of Physicians of Philadelphia; Vaccine Injury Compensation Programs; The History of Vaccines; updated Jan 2018; accessed March 2019

[10] WHO; Safety update of HPV vaccines; extract from GACVS meeting on 7-8 June 2017; accessed March 2019

Introduction

THIS BOOK IS NOT FICTION. It is a collection of stories about real people who trusted their physicians, government agencies and political representatives to protect the health and well-being of their children. It is a book about families who believed in vaccines. They 'knew' every vaccine had been thoroughly tested for safety and efficacy before being approved for public use. They had no reason to believe otherwise.

These families did not know HPV vaccines had been awarded fast-track status. They did not understand this status allowed HPV vaccines to be approved without having to undergo much of the safety testing typically required before approval of a drug, medical device, or vaccine.

These families did not have access to a critical piece of information from the FDA website which states:

Phase 4 trials are carried out once the drug or device has been approved by FDA during the Post-Market Safety Monitoring[11]

In short, these families had no idea they were voluntarily submitting their children to a phase 4 clinical trial. This is the best case scenario.

In some countries, HPV vaccines were government mandated. In these countries, people were virtually forced to participate in the world-wide phase 4 clinical trial without their knowledge or consent.

Until such time as HPV vaccination programs prove a reduction in cancer rates, this phase 4 trial will technically continue.

Until HPV vaccines are demonstrated to cause less harm than the cancers they are intended to prevent, the phase 4 clinical trial will still be underway.

Anyone who decides to use HPV vaccines before these two conditions are met is participating in a phase 4 clinical trial.

---

[11] US FDA; The Drug Development Process Step 3: Clinical Research; updated 01/04/2018; accessed March 2019

The families who submitted their personal stories for this book want to make sure others know the potential risks before they submit to participating in this huge medical experiment. They want people to have all the information necessary to make a free and informed decision regarding this particular medical intervention.

The families in this book do not want anyone else to have to travel the same road they were forced to take without being warned in advance.

It is their sincere hope that publishing these personal stories will help the world understand their children are not statistics. They are real people with real medical conditions which need treatment. They hope that allowing you to 'walk a mile' in their shoes will help you understand it is virtually impossible for all of their experiences to be coincidental.

Because the new symptoms are so diverse, they hope this book will inspire medical professionals to co-operate across multiple disciplines to develop treatment protocols to help their children regain at least some of their former abilities.

These families hope to inspire scientists to conduct research to find out why so many are being injured after HPV vaccines, so those most prone to adverse effects can be eliminated from future HPV vaccination programs.

These families hope government health officials will recognize the possibility that several new medical conditions might be associated with HPV vaccine administration and take measures to limit future devastation.

They want government health officials to recognize the possible risks associated with HPV vaccines as well as the promised, yet to be proven, benefits.

They want government health officials to provide complete and accurate information about HPV vaccines before injections are administered, the same informed consent which is currently required prior to any other medical procedure.

They want government health officials and politicians to stop trying to mandate medical interventions.

These families want to regain control of their healthcare choices. They no longer trust others to handle this responsibility for them and their families.

Read about their *Journeys from Trust to Tragedy* to find out why.

CHAPTER 1

North America

The United States

Gardasil was approved for use in the United States on June 8, 2006. Only one month later, the CDC recommended the HPV vaccine for all girls age 9-26 for the prevention of cervical cancer.[12] Due to aggressive lobbying, by March of 2007, 31 states were considering legislation that would have mandated Gardasil injections for middle school students.[13] Was this a direct result of the fact that Merck, the manufacturer of Gardasil, had hired PR expert Beverly J. Lybrand to design Gardasil's marketing campaign two years prior to FDA approval?

No one can argue the fact, Beverly Lybrand's Gardasil campaign produced results. According to an article in *ADWEEK,* Gardasil "generated $452.2 million in the first six months of 2007, with 54,000 prescriptions dispensed, per IMS Health, Plymouth Meeting, Pa. (total first-year sales were $628 million)."[14] Gardasil was off to a flying start with high expectations for the future.

---

[12] Houppert, Karen; Who's Afraid of Gardasil; 08 March 2007; The Nation; accessed March 2019

[13] Wang K, Chen Y, Ferguson SD, Leach RE (2013) HPV, the Scarlet Letters. Med J Obstet Gynecol 1(3): 1018.

[14] Applebaum, Michael; Beverly J. Lybrand, Merck Vaccines; ADWEEK; Oct 2007; accessed March 2019

In February 2007, *Pharmaceutical Executive* selected Gardasil for the '2006 Brand of the Year' award for creating a market out of thin air.[15] This was the first time this award had been given. Beverly Lybrand's 'Team Gardasil' had apparently exceeded everyone's expectations.

However, it did not take long before people began to express concerns over the safety and efficacy profile of Merck's new wonder drug. According to a 2008 article in the *New York Times,* Dr. Diane Harper, a professor of medicine at Dartmouth Medical School and a principal investigator on the clinical trials of both Gardasil and Cervarix, was concerned that Merck may have moved too fast in their efforts to promote Gardasil use. She stated:

"Merck lobbied every opinion leader, women's group, medical society, politicians, and went directly to the people — it created a sense of panic that says you have to have this vaccine now."[16]

What if the people who had been convinced to be 'One Less' would not have been 'One' in the first place? What if HPV vaccines caused more harm than the disease they intended to prevent? What if eliminating some types of HPV only led to a more virulent type filling in the gap? There were obviously many unanswered questions.

Despite the questions, Merck continued to apply for expanded uses for Gardasil. On October 16, 2009, Gardasil was approved for use in males, ages 9 through 26.[17] In December 2014, Merck gained FDA approval for their new Gardasil 9 HPV vaccine for use in girls age 9 through 26, and males age 9 through 26. Gardasil 9 contained antigens to 5 additional high-risk HPV types, so the promise was this new and improved Gardasil would eliminate a higher percentage of cancer diagnoses.

In October 2016, GlaxoSmithKline decided to discontinue sales of Cervarix in the United States.[18]

---

[15] Pharmaceutical Executive staff writer; Brand of the Year; 01 Feb 2007; PharmExec.com; accessed March 2019

[16] Rosenthal, Elisabeth; Drug Makers' Push Leads to Cancer Vaccines' Rise; Aug 2008; The New York Times; accessed March 2019

[17] CDC; FDA Licensure of Quadrivalent Human Papillomavirus Vaccine (HPV4, Gardasil) for Use in Males and Guidance from the Advisory Committee on Immunization Practices (ACIP); 28 May 2010; MMWR; accessed March 2019

[18] Hackett, Don Ward; Gardasil is the Last HPV Vaccine Standing; Precision Vaccinations; Oct 2016; accessed March 2019

By October 2018, Gardasil had been approved for males and females age 9 through 45.[19] Merck now had access to a very large cohort of potential customers with no competition. In spite of the obvious advantages, intensive lobbying efforts, a strong public awareness campaign, and a brilliant marketing strategy, less than half of United States teens are up to date on their recommended HPV vaccinations.[20]

According to the Infectious Diseases Society of America, "Only about 16 percent of U.S. adolescents have been fully vaccinated against human papillomavirus (HPV) by the time they turn 13, despite national recommendations that call for vaccination at 11 to 12 years of age."[21]

Perhaps the following personal accounts explain why.

---

[19] Ingram, Ian; FDA Oks HPV Vaccine for Adults Up to Age 45; Medpage Today; Oct 2018; accessed March 2019

[20] Women's Health Policy; The HPV Vaccine: Access and Use in the U.S.; The Kaiser Family Foundation; Oct 2018; accessed March 2019

[21] Infectious Diseases Society of America. "HPV vaccination rates remain critically low among younger adolescents in the U.S." ScienceDaily. ScienceDaily, 17 January 2019. accessed March 2019

I have 'one less' daughter

By Lisa Ericzon, Alexandria Bay, New York

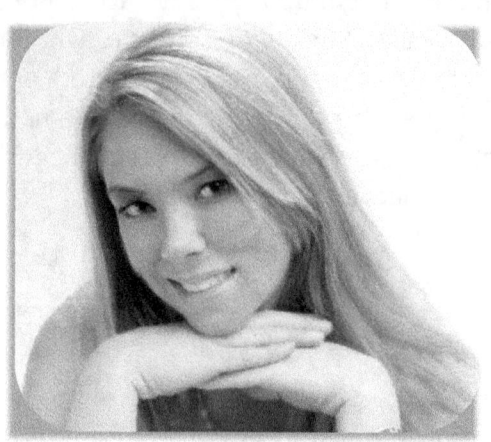

Jessie was delivered into this world by caesarean section on March 27, 1990. She weighed 7lbs 1 oz. Jess was a healthy baby and I was a happy Mom. So now we had a boy and a girl to make our family complete. Both of my kids were born in Watertown, New York approximately 25 miles from where I grew up. My husband John was a carpenter working at various jobs in the area, before going into business for himself. I was a stay at home mom and babysat for extra income. Before too long my husband joined the Carpenters Union and was driving many miles to certain jobs, because in our area union jobs were few and far between.

In September 1990 we moved to Rochester N.Y. which was 3 hours away from my family, where John was currently working on a good job. My Mom lived in Jacksonville Florida where I met John. After a year and a half in Rochester as a union carpenter my husband decided he wanted to become an over the road truck driver. So, against my wishes he went to school to become a tractor trailer driver. While he was in school, we decided that once he passed his road test and received his CDL we would move to Illinois where his family lived. So, in September of 1992 we moved to Ottawa Illinois where as soon as we unpacked the Truck John was on the road working for a carrier named Millis Transfer. He would be gone most of the week and home on the weekends, if I was lucky. So, I was raising my kids by myself for the most part with help from his family.

We lived in Illinois for 13 months before I had John move me back to Omar NY in October of 1993 so I could be close to my family and friends again. We had moved around a lot and I was determined to stay here and have my kids go to the same school their grandfather and I had.

So, when Jessie was 5 we bought my grandparent's house across the street from where we were renting an apartment. It was just across the road from my dad's dairy farm where my brother and I grew up.

Jessie and her brother Matt basically grew up on my dad's farm. We always helped whenever we could. If my brother and dad needed to be in the fields I would milk the cows and the kids were right there with me. I loved it. We had horses, so we always helped with the hay and many of the chores that came along with a dairy farm. I loved that my kids were getting this kind of life lesson. I think every kid should get the chance to grow up on a farm, it's very rewarding to see what hard work can achieve.

In January of 1998 the North Country was devastated by an ice storm and we were without power for 21 days. My husband was still driving tractor trailer and made it home the day after all the damage was done. We were able to get a generator to use for electricity and we burned wood so we didn't freeze. We had to borrow a tractor powered generator for the farm in order to do the milking. We were all ecstatic when they finally came to hook up the power 21 days after it was knocked out. Throughout this whole ordeal there was so much giving and generosity by everyone. Even the troops stationed at the Army Base of Fort Drum were making their rounds constantly to help where needed.

On Sunday, March 1998, at around 10:30 in the morning, I just happened to look out the window from my house across the road to the farm and saw a huge cloud of smoke. The cow barn was on fire! I called 911, grabbed the kids and jumped in the truck. When I got there my brother, my dad and a neighbor were just standing outside. It was already too late to save any livestock. The barn was a low wood structure and a free stall. All the cows had stampeded to the opposite end of the fire but there was so much smoke that most of them died of smoke inhalation. The main exit for the cows was at the other end of the barn where the fire was. Not a single cow or calf survived. We were devastated once again.

The barn was rebuilt the following year as a cover-all barn but with no milking parlor because dad was just going to raise heifers.

I am having a hard time with this part of the story, the part where I have to make my daughter real with only words. It's impossible for me to do. Not because I don't want to, but because I can't put into words my Jessie's spirit and life-force. The person she was becoming was the most amazing, compassionate, fun loving, good and moral person.

Both my kids went to the same school my dad and I did. It's a small school with K- 12 in the same building, so everyone knew everyone. The friends you made in kindergarten were still your friends when you graduated. We lived about 5 miles away so the kids had to ride the

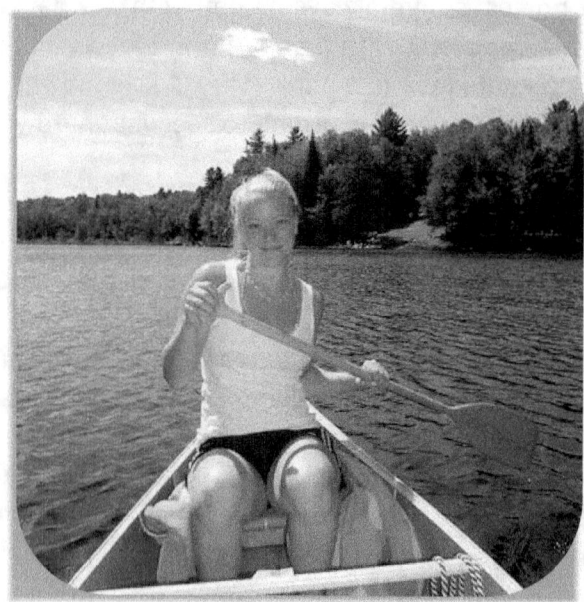

school bus. Jessie loved school.

Jess was involved in everything. When she was around 8 or 9 she started ice skating lessons and did that for a few years in the winter. Her brother Matt was into hockey. Since their father was on the road so much, it was always a challenge to get them to where they needed to be. Jess became

interested in basketball after a few years. She couldn't do both with all the practice involved, so basketball beat out ice skating. Jessie loved sports, softball was her favorite, tee ball was the beginning of that and from there it was all uphill I guess you could say.

Jess was a straight 'A' student involved in many clubs and activities. In her senior yearbook is a list of her accomplishments. J-V Basketball 7-10, Varsity Cheerleading 11-12, Softball 7-12, Band & Marching Band 7-10, Peer Leadership 9-12, Yearbook Club 1-4, Packs Peaks and Plants, Packs Paddle and Pollution. Spanish Club 9-12, Envirothon 11-12, Lions Club Scholar, National Honor Society, Prom Committee 3-4, Distance Learning 12. In that same yearbook each student has a famous "quote" and Jessie's quote was, **"The best things in life aren't things they're friends."**

Now that quote is on her headstone with the date of her death.

I was a Sunday school teacher, so Jess was brought up with a great sense of the Lord in her life. I was also a Brownie Leader then a Girl

Scout leader, so our garage was always filled with Girl Scout Cookies during the sale.

Jessie could never complain about being bored. She learned how to snowboard with her brother and the first time she tried water skiing she was able to get up out of the water and ski down the lake. Jessie excelled at everything. Echo Lake was our home away from home. In 1956 my grandparents, with the help of their 5 children, one of them being my mom, built a cabin in the Adirondacks on a small private lake. Jessie and Matt grew up there just like I did with my brother. Always swimming, hiking, canoeing, fishing, chopping wood and sitting by the fire. Our family always played cards in the evening before going to bed. Camp was always the best place to be with friends also, Jessie would bring her friends to camp and it was inevitable that they would have a shaving cream fight down at the beach, at the end they would all be lathered from head to toe with shaving cream.

In June of 2002 I left my husband and moved into my childhood home at the farm. Jessie came with me but her brother Matt stayed with his father.

In January of 2004 I met Tim at work, we were actually hired on the same day in August of 2002. Tim was hired for the hospital construction crew and I was hired to work in sterile processing. I never knew of him until my good friend who also worked at the hospital introduced us. When Jessie met Tim she immediately accepted him. There was never a cross word between the two of them, they became the best of friends.

In November 2004, Tim and I rented a house together and the 3 of us became a family. In February of 2006 Tim and I bought my grandparent's house, which is the same house Jessie and Matt grew up in. It will be the same house Jessie will die in also.

The few years the 3 of us had together were the best. We always had so much fun. It sounds like a lie when I say this but it was true; we never had any issues or fights between the 3 of us. We always got along. It was during this time that Jessie became old enough to get a job, so she got a summer job working at a small grocery and ice cream stand with her best friends. She would ride her bike to work and either Tim or I would go get her in the evening when she was done.

On July 29 2005, my brother and his friend had just finished work and were on their way home after cashing their checks at the bank. No one knows what happened but his friend just drove off the road and hit a telephone pole killing both of them instantly, just a quarter mile from where Jessie was working.

Now as I think back on that time, I feel that God was preparing me for what would happen when Jessie passed. I felt I knew what to do with all the arrangements for Jessie because I had just gone through it with my brother. I also now know what my Mom went through after losing her child. That's all I will say about that time of our lives.

In April of 2007 Jessie was put on Yasmine birth control which was prescribed by the doctor to hopefully help control acne that Jess was having a problem with. During this visit the doctor mentioned Jessie getting the Gardasil vaccine. We had never heard of this vaccine and wanted more info on it. We were told by the doctor that it would prevent cervical cancer in young girls Jessie's age when they get older.

I said no at the time and was given a brochure on the Gardasil vaccine to take home and look at. In the brochure it explained about the Human Papilloma Virus or HPV and that the possible side effects were pain, swelling, itching, and redness at the injection site, fever, nausea and dizziness. That was it for side effects at this time.

I remember the T.V. commercials about Gardasil, have your daughter become "ONE LESS" to get cervical cancer in her future. My license plate for my car now says "ONELESS' but it's because I now have one less daughter.

On July 16, 2007, we went for a re-check on Jess's acne and decided at this time to go ahead and get Jessie vaccinated against cervical cancer. How could I not want to protect my daughter against getting cervical cancer in the future? At the time it was a no brainer to me. Jessie wasn't afraid of needles and the first of three vaccinations was uneventful.

The summer of 2007 was spent focusing on colleges Jessie would possibly attend. Because she wanted to become a state trooper she would have to take courses geared toward that, so she decided to go for psychology. We took Emilia with us when we went to visit Plattsburgh State University in upstate New York. We took advantage of the opportunity to go camping and hiking at Ausable Chasm during the same trip. Both girls loved it there so much, they decided to apply to Plattsburgh along with a couple other colleges including Cazenovia, which is where my mother and her family are from.

On September 17, 2007 Jessie received her second Gardasil vaccination with no problems. I have an entry in my journal on October 23, saying, "Jessie is complaining of dizziness, headaches, muscle and joint aches and pains and being tired."

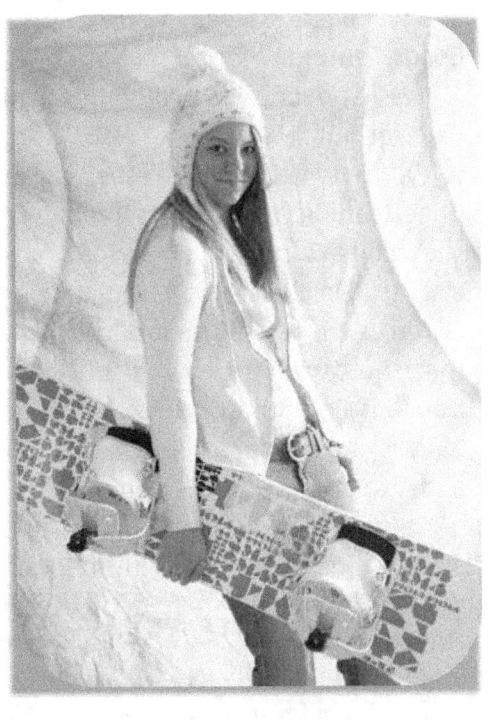

At the time I didn't really think much of this because Jessie was always on the go with everything and this was the first time I had heard her complaining.

Jessie's senior year was of course exciting and hectic and stressful, but Jess wouldn't have it any other way. She was always going at the speed of light. But she kept complaining of headaches and her joints hurting. We thought we could explain her muscle and joint pain because she started cheerleading practice and was a base so she was the one throwing and catching the other girls. The headaches were another story though. She was having those more frequently.

So, on November 20th, we went back to the doctor to have him check out her headaches. The doctor could find no reason at the time for her headaches, he said it was probably because she was a senior and she is under a lot of stress lately. If she feels a headache coming on just take some Tylenol. Neither the doctor, nor I ever thought it could be the Gardasil vaccine. At this visit Gardasil was never even mentioned.

So here we are into November and December with Basketball games and Cheerleading competitions, the Christmas Ball and parties. In December Jessie wrote a letter to the local State Trooper Barracks requesting a ride-along with one of the Troopers. After signing paperwork and permission slips Jessie was given a date of February 16, 2008 for her State Trooper Ride-Along. She was so excited and nervous.

January 2008, the beginning of a new year, Jessie will be graduating in a few months. She has been accepted at Plattsburgh State University and will begin classes in August. Her class is going to Disney World and Epcot Center in Florida on March 6th for their Senior Trip. Life is good!

Jessie never got to go on her Senior Trip. Jessie's cap and gown were paid for but Jessie never got to graduate with her best friends.

February 2008, Basketball is over for the season and no more Cheerleading. Jess can now focus on the upcoming Softball season and she wants to pitch this season. Jessie is also taking Distance Learning classes which are offered through JCC, a community college in Watertown, just 30 miles from Lafarge Ville. Extra credits are earned that she can apply toward her college credits for next fall. Valentines Dance is Feb 8th and Jess and all her friends are going as a group. Feb 15th is the school's Winter Carnival with all kinds of games and prizes and a ton of fun for the community.

Saturday, February 16, 2008 Jessie gets to go on her Trooper ride-along. When she comes in the door after her ride-along she is ecstatic, this is what she wants to do for sure! Jessie got to ride with the K-9-unit, Officer Poggi and his German shepherd, Ram. What a fantastic time she had and officer Poggi was so nice!

February 18 through February 22, school was off for winter break. A lot of the students and teachers went to warmer climates during this break. Jessie's best friend Emilia and her good friend Amanda went to Amanda's father in Connecticut. We stayed home during this time but Jessie had Distance Learning classes to attend at JCC on Wednesday and Friday. She and her classmates would ride the bus to JCC for the class which they would normally take in her own school, but because school was closed for Winter Break that week they had to go to JCC on the bus. During this week also, school allowed the girls to come to open gym so they could practice pitching for the upcoming season with the help of their coaches.

February 20th, Wednesday, after Jessie's Distance Learning class and Open Gym she met me at the doctor's office for her third and final Gardasil vaccination around 5pm. The next day Jess went to Open Gym for help from the coaches with her pitching. When Tim and I got home from work, (we work at the same hospital so we can ride together) Jessie was on the couch resting as she was tired.

Later that night Jess and I sat on the couch together and were doing a Sudoku Puzzle on her lap top. She complained again of a headache, something she hadn't done for the last couple of weeks. There was a spot behind her left ear which she complained about before, was bothering her again. I told her to take some Tylenol before she went to bed and hopefully she would feel better in the morning. She had to meet the bus at school in order to ride to JCC in the morning for her Distance Learning class.

About 9pm I gave her a kiss goodnight and told her that I loved her and went to bed. At 5am, on Friday, February 22, 2008 when Tim and I left for work, Jess was sleeping as usual.

I play the scenario of what could have happened that morning in my head over and over again. I picture this in my mind:

> *Jess gets out of bed around 9:15 or 9:30, you see Jess didn't like to get up too early. She knows nobody is home so she comes downstairs in what she slept in, her heather grey t-shirt that says 'SENIOR 2008' on the front and 'DONE' on the back. I think back on how ironic it is that her shirt says 'DONE' on the back. The lettering on her shirt is a light blue almost the color of her eyes. Jess goes into the bathroom, turns on the light and shuts the door. I picture her standing in front of the mirror looking at her face and sticking out her tongue. Maybe she fixed the ponytail that her beautiful thick blond hair was in. After using the toilet, she stands up and turns around to flush. Something is wrong, Oh My God she feels terrified! She doesn't know what is happening! What went on in those few seconds before she collapsed?? "MOM! MOM!" she says. But I'm not there. I'M NOT THERE!! Jessie died all by herself with me not there to be with her when she needed me the most. I never got to say GOODBYE TO JESS. I NEVER GOT TO SAY I LOVE YOU SO MUCH.*

I truly believe I could have saved her if I was at home that morning. That day will haunt me for the rest of my life. The things I remember about that day are so vivid in my mind and so unbelievable. I still can't believe she is gone.

At school, the bus waited and waited for Jessie. Someone called her cell phone a couple of times I'm sure. The bus left for JCC without her and since it wasn't a regular school day I never got a phone call at work telling me Jessie never showed up. I think about that now, and wonder what would have happened if I had received a call. I would have kept trying to call her from work. When I never got an answer, I probably would have called my Dad to go and see if she was even home. He

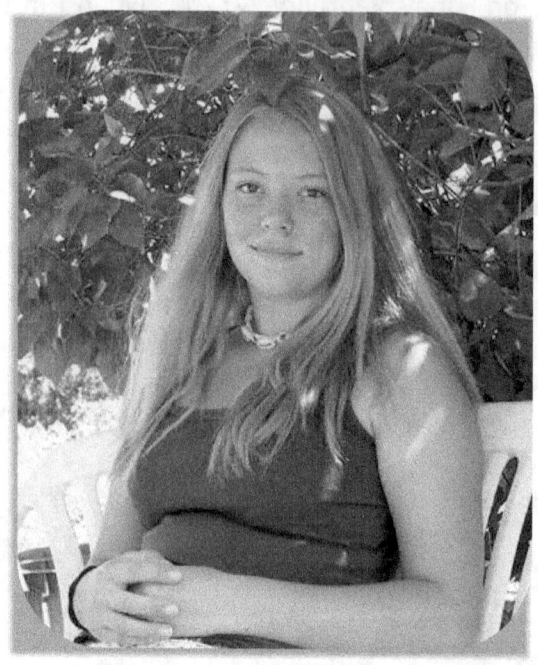

would have seen her Jeep in the driveway and would have gone in the house to see if she was OK. I believe things happen for a reason, there was a reason for no phone call from school that day. God didn't want my Dad to find Jessie dead on the bathroom floor. Instead it was me who found her.

I won't go into much detail about this moment in my life, but I can tell you that it was indescribable, something I have a hard time even putting words to. My brain went into overload and everything I was thinking at that moment was so unreasonable and unreal. I knew she was dead, but I wanted the ambulance to get here so someone would give her CPR. Her skin was cold, but I thought that was from getting out of the shower and you feel cold. When I moved her, her breath escaped a little and I thought she was alive. At the same time I knew she wasn't. Jessie's eyes were barely open and I could see the blue of her iris, as if she were watching me. I lay my head on her chest and begged her to forgive me for not being here for her. It wasn't real, this couldn't be real.

Tim met the first Trooper to arrive in the driveway. The Ambulance arrived at the same time. The EMT's were turned away because they would not have been able to do anything. Tim had been a member of a volunteer fire department and he knew that there was no help for

Jessie. He had seen this type of thing before. Our home was filling with Troopers and I remember a female Trooper coming to kneel on the floor by the bathroom door. She was blonde and had her hair in a ponytail like Jessie's and she was very young. She starts speaking to me very softly and compassionately. She tells me that they will take care of Jessie now and maybe I would like to come and sit for a minute while she asked me some questions.

They had to treat our home as a crime scene now, although I never thought of it at the time. Tim says that I mentioned that Jessie had the Gardasil vaccination 2 days ago but I don't remember saying that. It's funny how the brain acts when you're in shock. As Tim and I are answering questions the phone rings.

Tim can tell by the caller ID that it's Emilia, Jessie's best friend. When Tim answered the phone, Emilia was hysterical and wanted to know if it was true what she had just found out. She had seen through a text message that Jessie was dead. Tim told her that Jessie was gone and then I'm not sure what else was said because he walked into the office.

He came back a minute later saying that she knew before he told her. One of Jessie's classmates heard the call go out over the scanner about a teenage girl at the Ericzon residence that was unresponsive. He sent a mass text message to all his friends and Emilia received that message while she was in Connecticut with Amanda.

After the Officer finished asking me questions, she said that they had to do an investigation and I could not be there, did I have some place to go? So, I told her I would be across the road at the farm. The feeling of never seeing my daughter alive again was so overwhelming it's indescribable. I could not believe this was happening. I was having a nightmare I could not wake up from. I was leaving Jessie alone with a houseful of Troopers and I would never see her face again.

That afternoon was a blur. I do remember vividly my terror of having to call my mom, my son Matt and his father to let them know what happened. I couldn't bring myself to call my Mom because just two and a half years earlier, I had to call her to tell her that her son, my brother, was killed in a car accident. So now it's déja vu all over again. So, my Step-mom called her.

On Saturday, February 23, 2008, the Coroner called with the results of Jessie's autopsy report. It concluded that she had died of unknown causes. He could find no reason for Jessie's death. Then, I remembered she had had her Gardasil vaccination just 40 hours before she died. He said to me that he had never heard of any negative feedback on this vaccine, of course her toxicology report was going to take a while for the results. He had even sent a sample of Jessie's brain tissue to a Neuropathologist in Syracuse.

For the next week Tim and I stayed at the farm as I could not go back to our home just yet. But Tim went home to use the computer to do research on Gardasil. When he brought me copies of some of the articles on Gardasil I was BLOWN AWAY by what I read. It seems that Gardasil was killing some of the young women who are being vaccinated with it. I knew right then that it was Gardasil that killed Jessie. I was so shocked and horrified by what I read, and it was only the tip of the iceberg as we would find out over time.

July 2008, you can't sue Merck or any other Big Pharma for killing your daughter. You have to find a lawyer who deals in vaccine injury cases. In July of 2008, I wasn't even thinking of any kind of litigation. I had been speaking to Susan Edelman, a reporter from the N.Y. Post, who was doing an article on Jessie and Gardasil. I asked her questions and she told me about the Vaccine Injury Compensation Program. Susan had been speaking to a lawyer who specializes in vaccine injury about Gardasil.

On Sunday, July 20th 2008 the N.Y. post printed the article about Jessie. Basically, I was saying that the Gardasil vaccine had killed my daughter. At 11am someone from CBS called and wanted me to be on *The Early Show* to tell my story about Jessie and Gardasil. They wanted me to come to New York City tomorrow! At 1pm, they were calling me to find out where the closest airport was. At 4pm they called me back to tell me CBS was going to wait and do some more research before going ahead with the story.

Since that first N.Y. Post article I have been interviewed on the radio, my local newspaper, the local television station and many more ways. My mom has also been very involved in trying to get the word out about Gardasil. She has also been on the radio and newspapers in her area. So along with all the media and the web, Jessie's story was getting out there.

We were also hearing of other girls losing their lives to this vaccine.

Right about this time, with all the media focused on Jessie, Tim came to me one evening with the copy of an e-mail from Erin Brockovich. Yes, THE Erin Brockovich that the movie about PG & E focused on. Tim was doing research as usual and was looking up lawyers and just happened to somehow contact Erin. She just said that if there was anything she could do to help that she was available for any questions. I still wasn't ready to consider any kind of litigation.

Susan Edelman e-mailed me to tell me that a college girl mysteriously died not long after her Gardasil vaccine. Susan wanted to know if I would like to talk to this other mother. So, I gave permission to Susan to give this person my information. After receiving an e-mail from Emily and getting to finally talk to her on the phone we both realized that we were going through the same thing. Both of our daughters died after their Gardasil vaccine. They both had the same symptoms before they passed and now I wasn't alone in this anymore. We spoke often on the phone just to see how we were both doing. We kept hearing about other girls who had died after their Gardasil vaccine. All these girls were experiencing the same tiredness, achy muscles, headaches, and dizziness as Jessie and Christina.

In September of 2008, I actually spoke to Erin Brockovich on the phone and asked her questions about finding a lawyer who could help us. Erin said at that time there were over 13,000 VAERS reports about death or adverse reactions to the Gardasil vaccine. Erin put me in touch with an assistant for Girardi and Keese, who I retained in December of 2008.

On May 11, 2009 I received a letter from Girardi and Keese saying they will not file or pursue claims or lawsuits against Merck, stating, *"We have concluded that meeting our burden of demonstrating causation poses a far too difficult factual hurdle."*

After receiving another letter from another law firm that was similar, this firm suggested going to Conway, Homer and Chin-Caplin from Boston, this firm specializes in the Vaccine Injury Compensation Program. A government program where you have to have a special master who decides your case and not a regular court.

In September of 2009, I retained the services of Conway, Homer and Chin-Caplin to represent Jessie through me to prove that Gardasil was what caused her death. Little did I know it would take 6 long grief-filled years to get a ruling on our case.

After years of waiting and waiting and going nowhere, there just wasn't enough info out there and Merck wasn't parting with any. In April of 2013 on a whim, my lawyer sent slides of Jessie's tissue samples to a new neuropathologist they had been using for pediatric cases. He found something in Jessie's slide samples that Jessie's original autopsy didn't see. Vasculitis of the brain not caused by a virus.

The respondent's expert witness also looked at Jessie's samples and this expert agreed that he did see vasculitis on the brain. One way to get vasculitis is if you have a virus and I know Jessie didn't have a virus at the time. So, my lawyer talked about the next step and that would be that in similar cases the special master is encouraging settlement or if it went to trial they would be booking cases into January 2014.

In June of 2013, the Respondent (the Department of Health or Health and Human Services) made me an offer to settle for $ 20,000.00. What a slap in the face! So, I told my lawyer to proceed to a hearing. The hearing date was set for January 22 & 23, 2014.

November 18 the Canary Party released on you tube the "Not a Coincidence" video with many of the girls and their moms talking about the Gardasil vaccine and that it is Not a coincidence that all these girls are dying or getting sick from this vaccine.

January 16, 2014, I get another offer from HHS, this time it is $50,000. They said this was their best and final offer. I said no to this again and to proceed to a hearing. My lawyer tells me Jessie's case is very unusual that it's usually infants or old people who are dying from vaccines. With Gardasil there are no established cases and I told my lawyer that Jessie's case may be the first.

On January 27th 2014, my lawyer calls to tell me the testimony went well. It was all done by teleconference. No decision was made, just evidence was presented. Both neuropathologists agreed they saw the vasculitis in Jessie's brain. Our side said it was caused by the Gardasil vaccine and their side said it was caused by an infection. HHS is overwhelmed with many cases and my lawyer feels that the Special Masters are pressured to 'deny'. This case could drag on for another 1 or 2 years.

June 2014, HHS is still saying that the Vasculitis is caused by Mycoplasma Pneumonia, it's a lung infection sometimes called walking pneumonia. Jessie wasn't sick when she passed and I knew this but now they have to prove it. So, the Special Master can order the CDC to do testing on Jessie's lung tissue, both experts are ordered to do a report on Mycoplasma Pneumonia. My lawyer feels like this case is being treated like a criminal case where guilt has to be proven beyond a reasonable doubt. There will be a conference scheduled for July 22 where they will discuss the findings of the expert witnesses.

August 5, 2014, my lawyer says this case has taken so many twists and turns that she has never seen before. Now the Special Master wants to go through mediation, which means they want to bring in a 3rd party to hear the evidence and make suggestions. Both my lawyer and HHS have to agree to the mediation. August 20, 2014, HHS had decided against mediation. Now the Special Master has the next call. The attorney for HHS has thrown another offer to us of $15,000. REALLY? I rejected the offer immediately.

Sept 23, 2014, the court ordered further testing. If I refuse, the case will be dismissed. So I told my lawyer that this is in God's hands and I trust in the Lord - so we will go ahead with the testing.

January 26, 2015, the results of the CDC testing on Jessie's tissue for Mycoplasma Pneumonia have come back negative. I knew she wasn't sick at all and this finally proves it to HHS. This knocks the legs out from under the HHS case. Now a report has to be filed with the court; then it's up to the Special Master what happens next. I'm so scared they will find something else to argue against.

March 10th 2015, my lawyer called to say that the respondent has approached her with another settlement offer, she said she was very shocked by this. She feels that the Special Master has pushed for a settlement so she doesn't have to make the decision. HHS has offered to settle Jessie's case for $175,000. The maximum death benefit through this program is 250,000. But, that is if you win the case. After a few counter offers, I settled. I won't disclose the amount I received for Jessie's death, but I will say it was very close to the max amount.

I felt like I was responsible for Jessie's death and now here I am taking money for it. I can't describe the feelings that went through me except it was all guilt and feeling like I let Jessie down in every way by not taking it all the way to the end. I was scared that all the waiting and hard work would be for absolutely nothing if I would have lost. So, I caved and settled out of court basically. I can't say anything more about this, it makes my stomach sink to know that I didn't follow through for Jessie.

So, this is Jessie's story, a very short version of her life and my struggles against Merck, a Pharmaceutical company who cares for money more than people's lives. A company who fast tracked the clinical trials. A company who wouldn't even listen to people who worked closely with this vaccine, who told them of the dangers. There is so much more that could be written, sometimes I feel I could write a book of my own with everything that has transpired since Jessie's death, the good and the bad. Even out of all the pain and grief there are so many things that were unbelievable and I know God had a hand in it, and that is the only way I can explain some of the experiences I have had.

I feel I have won a very small battle against a giant. I do feel by the combined efforts of all the people who are involved with this struggle we have made a difference. Gardasil is hardly ever referred to as Gardasil. I believe it got such a bad name that Merck had to change the name to the HPV Vaccine.

I hope people will read this book and make the decision not to vaccinate. I hope they will not trust their doctor with their child's life like I did and that they will research every aspect of any drug that is put into their bodies. I wish I had done so for Jessie's sake, she would be here now if I had.

Gardasil will not destroy us

By Leah Marsh, Utah

When Emily was 12-years- old, she was a happy full of life girl. She loved to read and go to school. She was a straight 'A' student and was also taking honor classes. She would read about 4 books a month. Emily and I would both read the same book, then discuss what we had read. We had started reading the Michael

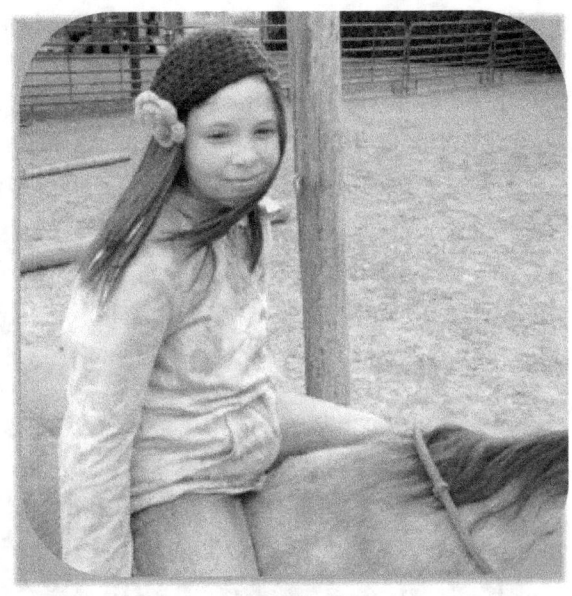

Vey series when she got sick. We never did finish the books. Her other passions were playing the piano and riding horses. She was an amazing piano player. I never had to remind her to practice. She loved playing the theme to Star Wars. Every morning before school she would play the piano. It was the best part of the morning.

She loved to help her younger siblings with their homework. She loved to play pranks on her brother and sister. She would check books out of the library on practical jokes to get new ideas.

She was the type of girl that if she saw someone at school that didn't have a friend she would make the effort to make them feel accepted.

In 2015 Emily received 2 shots of the HPV vaccine Gardasil. Within a week Emily started to complain about her eyesight. She said that she was seeing black dots in her vision. I took her to an eye doctor where we discovered she had optical neuritis in her right eye. She was put on high-dose steroids and we thought all was well.

On December 9, 2015, Emily was practicing the piano, when her brother came and got me saying Emily was doing something odd. I ran to Emily and found her having a seizure. I had to call 911, as she was not coming out of it. They did a spinal tap and told us to go home. She ended up having more seizures and she was put on anti-seizure medications that didn't help.

By December 26th, Emily could no longer talk or really walk. The seizures continued. She was admitted to the hospital where she would stay for close to 3 months. The left side of her brain is inflamed and she has lesions as well. She had around 4 spinal taps, brain biopsy and 15 treatments of plasmapheresis. Nothing helped my sweet girl. The brain biopsy revealed that her T cells were attacking her brain.

I had to sit in the hospital and watch my daughter disappear. The

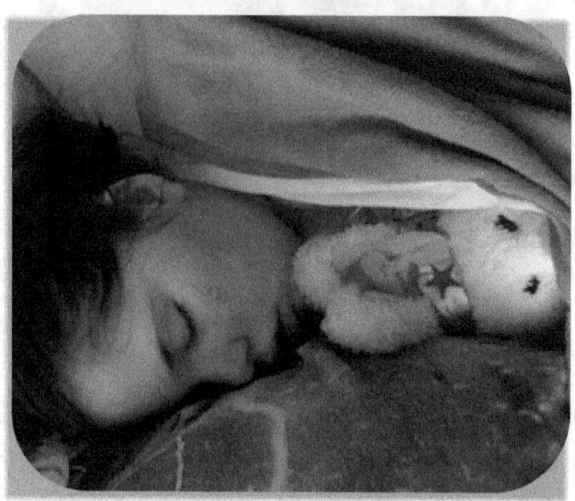

right side of her body was no longer working very well, and twitched all the time. Her mouth twitched so bad that she could not eat or drink very well. She would frequently choke on water.

Before she was released from the hospital, doctors told me there was no hope for my daughter and that I had to accept this as Emily's 'new normal'. After she was released from the hospital, we had to find ways to deal with her new medical conditions on our own.

Emily could no longer function in a public school, so I was forced to put her on a home school program. Since being abandoned by the traditional medical professionals, we have been seeing a homeopathic doctor in Idaho. We go every week and have been doing so for about 7 months. She does IV therapy and neuro- therapy. Since we started the homeopathic treatments, there have been some improvements. She can now eat and drink without choking. Her mouth twitch stopped and we have been able to reduce her seizure medications.

I am so glad we refused to accept what the traditional doctors said to us. We are so thankful to our homeopathic doctor in Idaho for treating us so well – it has been such a blessing.

When I was asked how I saw my daughter's future – my response was:

- I know my daughter is going to get better.
- I know my daughter will walk again.
- I know my daughter will talk again.

And I know we are going to go to that hospital and prove to the doctors that they were wrong when they said that Emily would never recover. Emily will show them how well she has recovered by playing the piano for them.

A mother, with faith on her side, has more power to overcome the worst possible nightmares that took over her life following Emily's vaccinations with Gardasil.

Gone, not forgotten

By Kathleen Berrett (Colton's Mom), Utah, USA

Gardasil catastrophically took away my son Colton Berrett's happy amazing life, leaving him paralyzed from the neck down and ventilator dependent February 2014.

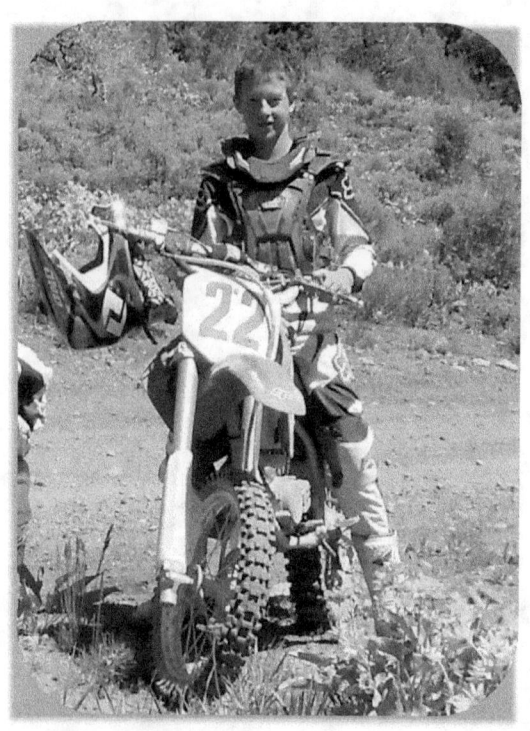

Colton Berrett was born a happy, healthy, energetic boy on March 13, 2000. Growing up he was full of life, excited to learn new things and always had a smile on his face. He enjoyed participating in sports and going camping with our family. He loved to play baseball, basketball, snow ski, ride a scooter, skateboard and bike. He enjoyed water sports and loved diving, jumping and swimming in the water. He was often found running around the neighborhood with friends playing air soft gun wars. However, his greatest passion was motocross. He started riding a motorcycle at the age of 6 and progressed through the years to ride as well as his dad.

Colton was known as a very active and healthy boy. In fact, many of our friends commented on how lucky he was because 'he never gets sick'. The only illness he had ever dealt with in his life was the occasional common cold when the seasons changed.

Colton was maturing into a handsome, strong, athletic and independent young man. During the summer of 2013, he loved wearing tank tops to show off his muscles. He enjoyed trying to impress girls, taking selfies and posting them on social media to get the most likes possible.

Little did we know that this amazing life was going to be tragically and drastically altered in February of 2014.

As a mother you strive to do whatever you can to keep your kids healthy and safe. When our doctor recommended Colton receive the Gardasil vaccination series to protect him from various types of cancer, we didn't hesitate. After each shot, his arm was extra sore and felt like he had a fever in it. They were by far the most painful vaccinations he'd ever had.

On February 1, 2014, Colton received the third and final dose of the series. It takes 2 weeks for your body's immune system to respond to a vaccine. Like clockwork Colton woke up 13 days later with a bad neck ache that got progressively worse over the next couple of days.

Despite still being in pain, he was still excited to get out and ride the new motorcycle he had received at Christmas for the first time. During the ride, he began to get very weak and went straight to bed when he got home dirty clothes and all. He stayed there all night and throughout the next day.

Late Sunday evening, he began to tell me he wanted his water cup placed on his left side so he could pick it up. He said he was having a hard time lifting his right arm. His right arm was becoming paralyzed first since it was the one the vaccination was administered in. He had tried to rise onto his elbow in order to take some pain medicine and get a drink, but when he did that he suddenly flopped back saying he couldn't hold his head up and it made him nauseous when he tried to sit up. It was so late he asked if we could take him to Instacare first thing in the morning if he wasn't feeling better.

Fortunately, Colton woke up! However, the tragic events of becoming completely paralyzed were beginning to unfold. He could still not hold his head up or move his right arm. His dad had to hold his head upright in order to walk him out to the car.

Colton was only thirteen years old when he was admitted to Primary Children's Hospital in Salt Lake City on February 17, 2014. This hospitalization lasted a total of 88 days.

The neurologist trying to figure out what could be causing this mysterious paralysis asked many questions regarding Colton's health because the tests they were running weren't showing signs of any viral infection. So, he started back tracking and asked if Colton had been sick or if anything different had happened during the last couple weeks. I told the doctor he hadn't been sick and the only thing different in his life was that he'd had the Gardasil vaccine. The doctor's jaw dropped and he immediately said he'd report it to VAERS.

When the MRI imaging came back it showed inflammation in Colton's spinal cord that extended from C-1 (the top vertebra in the spinal column) to the cauda equine (A bundle of nerve roots that branch off the lower spine). As the day went on, he also began losing function down his left arm.

While in the emergency room, Colton told his dad with tears and fear in his eyes, "Dad, I don't want to be paralyzed!"

This literally was Colton's only 'complaint' through his journey with TM, Transverse Myelitis. A year later, his diagnosis was changed to AFM. (**AFM**) Acute flaccid myelitis is a rare condition of the nervous system that causes the muscles and reflexes of the body to weaken. Symptoms are a sudden onset of arm or leg weakness and loss of muscle tone and reflexes.

Shortly after his MRI, it was determined that he was going to stop being able to breathe on his own so he should be intubated. We didn't take into consideration how this procedure would alter our ability to communicate with Colton.

Over the next 4 days, the paralysis crept all the way down to his toes. He was now ventilator dependent and a complete quadriplegic. He couldn't do anything but raise or scrunch his eyebrows to answer yes or no questions as we tried figuring out what we could do to make him more comfortable.

He spent the next 3 weeks in the pediatric intensive care unit fighting for his life, as well as trying to recover from the surgery performed for a permanent tracheotomy and a feeding tube insertion.

He was uncomfortable and frustrated having to use only his eyebrows to express his emotions, pain and discomfort. Due to the nerve pain in his legs we constantly had to reposition him to try and get him comfortable. He was fitted for a TLSO brace, we called a turtle shell, and AFO braces. Each day he had to be strapped into each brace as well as a cervical brace to support his head in order to start his therapies while in the hospital.

Colton's rigorous daily routine began. In addition to all his personal care, such as bathing, dressing, and strapping all of his braces on, he had to do preparatory stretches, physical therapy, occupational therapy and respiratory therapy. Respiratory therapy consists of a cough assist program completed every 4 hours to keep his lungs clear. All of this would have to be performed by nurses or his parents for the rest of his life. Colton's hospital days were very strenuous. In spite of everything, he woke up each day with powerful motivation and a strong determination to get better while sporting an infectious smile that made everyone fall in love with him.

Colton celebrated his 14th birthday in the hospital. Colton had been an impressive individual and now he was embarrassed to have to be seen in his debilitated state by his friends and peers who came to visit.

Rob and I were trained to handle everything required for Colton's care including the special jobs involved because of his need to be on the ventilator so we could take him home. It was overwhelming and frightening. Colton was so trusting and had such confidence in our ability to perform the tasks required for his survival. He was the best Patient!

After a month-and-a-half of being completely paralyzed, Colton did a miraculous thing, he began to raise his feet 6 inches off the bed. We had been told that function regained during the first year would be what his new normal life would be.

This motivated him even more to work as hard as he did. Colton made baby steps of improvements throughout the next two months in the Hospital. Finally, on May 15, 2014, we were able to bring him home.

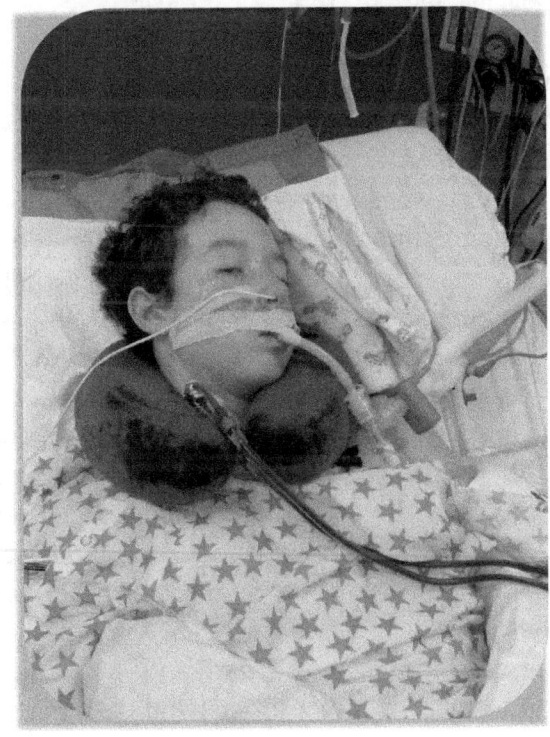

Our new routine at home began. Colton spent many hours 4 days a week travelling long distances after school to physical therapy and doctor appointments trying and helping him to regain strength in his extremities. Though it was exhausting, we did this for the rest of his life.

He relearned how to walk, eat food, and use only half his left arm while continuing to gain strength in his core. Tragically he would never regain head or neck control, use his right arm or have the ability to breathe without his ventilator, aka life support. The ventilator was a literal ball and chain. He could not carry it, so someone had to carry it for him. He was forced to have constant care 24/7.

We had to open our home to nurses that came to help relieve us of the strain of running a family while caring for Colton's immediate needs. Nurses also escorted him to school every day from the beginning of his freshman year through half his senior year.

Compassionate, caring Colton didn't like feeling he was a burden to us. He would often apologize to us because of his medical needs. It broke our hearts that he felt bad for us.

He was so patient and understanding. He never complained if we pulled too hard on his vent cord choking him or took him off the vent when he wasn't ready. Sometimes I wouldn't hear him call for help in the middle of the night. He never had a cross word to say. Nor did he blame me for allowing him to have the vaccination. That guilt however, I will live with for the rest of my life.

Colton's new physical appearance was very interesting and would attract stares from people of all ages. Colton despised this attention yet he still never complained. He would just smile and shock people by saying 'Hi'.

Colton was always quick to crack a joke and make you laugh. He had awesome friends at school, but never felt like he could enjoy the dating life because he couldn't drive or go anywhere by himself.

Great disappointment struck again when surgery to help him breathe without a ventilator failed. Now he couldn't get rid of his ball and chain ventilator. His hopes and dreams of ever being an independent adult were shattered. He would never get to date, never drive or get a job since he couldn't do these activities without assistance with his ventilator and a friend carrying it.

He continued to work very hard at physical therapy so he could learn to breathe without the ventilator for periods of time. The only muscles that would function were his intercostals (muscle groups situated between the ribs that create and move the chest wall primarily used to assist the breathing process) and right peck. Being off the ventilator for extended periods of time was straining on his body and made him tired, yet he still managed to do it for an hour or two a day. This gave him a little bit of independence while at home.

Colton's healthy, active life had been ripped from him and we mourned with him. The loss of each one of his abilities and all of the events that should've taken place during his precious teenage years caused an indescribable sense of sadness and grief for the entire family.

Each of us handled our grief privately. For Colton, we did our best to maintain our family's usual adventurous nature. Our goal was to keep him active by getting him out camping and riding. Adapting to Colton's needs, we completed 26 camping adventures during those three years. We had to run a generator all night in order to power his equipment and charge his ventilator batteries so everything would function properly the following day.

Instead of a motorcycle we bought him a Polaris RZR (side by side ATV) that he learned to pilot with great skill using only half his left arm from the elbow to his hand, and his legs to steer and drive. He loved the ability to go fast, whipping donuts and spraying sand and dust on those near him.

He also had a recumbent trike that we adapted for left hand use with a basket on the back for his ventilator. He used it to cruise around the neighborhood to enjoy a little freedom from constant care. It was a great way to hang out with his best friend, giving him a break from watching television or playing the Xbox.

Colton participated in adaptive sports including snow skiing, sailing and even horseback riding for therapy. Although these activities seemed fun they were hard on his body physically and didn't live up to the action he had been accustomed to before the Gardasil injections. His 'ball and chain' ventilator made all of his favorite activities simply fond memories. Still, he did not complain.

During an interview with the Vaxxed crew, he fought back the tears as he tried to explain how hard it was to be someone that had to just sit on the sidelines now. His very next statement was that he was getting used to it so it's not so bad. (Like I said before, he truly never complained.)

Colton made it to his senior year in high school. He had worked very hard to get good grades. He did have the help of his nurses, but they were really just Colton's glorified pack mules. The nurses helped him get from classroom to classroom.

During this year, Colton's friends were all growing up and becoming young independent adults. Everyone around him seemed to be getting jobs, dating and talking about what their futures held for them. Soon they would be graduating from high school and going their separate ways. Many were making plans to serve missions for the Church of Jesus Christ of Latter-day Saints. This was a dream Colton had nurtured his whole life. He felt like this opportunity wouldn't be attainable in his paralyzed condition. It must have been terribly hard for him to know he would not be able to fulfill this dream, but he still did not complain.

Colton knew he was loved. He also knew what living a healthy life was like prior to the devastating side effects he experienced after Gardasil. He despised the idea of remaining dependent on others for the rest of his life. Air being forced down his throat via a tube hooked to his neck by a trach was a grueling experience in itself; let alone having to try and deal with the consequences of being trapped in a body that won't work for you. Having little hope of some semblance of recovering his normal life took its toll on him.

He felt like a burden to the family. What he didn't realize was how much we loved him for who he was and that we stood in awe of the strength he had to endure the challenges he faced with such faith and dignity.

Colton had been cared for 24/7 for almost 4 yrs. He grew up not having his own personal space. He was always with parents, a sibling, or a nurse by his side to take care of him.

On January 5, 2018, Colton had been smiling and happy at school. He'd made plans for the next day with his nurse. Dad and brother were heading off to a motorcycle event while Mom and sister went to a movie. It had been typical for Colton to decline going out in public, especially when it was cold.

This evening we decided to give the nurse the night off and I would tend to Colton's needs when I returned home. Colton being a teenager, I felt he should be allowed some alone time, even though he hadn't asked.

Colton had never experienced any serious medical emergencies since he'd been discharged from the hospital, so it gave me a little comfort knowing it was time to start allowing him a bit of freedom from having someone constantly hovering near him. We had never left him all alone, but knowing he could call us or a friend, we figured it would be all right for a couple hours. He asked me to put a movie in for him which he watched most of.

When we returned from our separate activities, Colton wasn't in his regular chair so we thought he was being his typical self, quietly hiding and waiting to scare us. That was not the case.

Our hearts sank as we found that in a moment of weakness our son had decided it would be better if he removed himself from this life and his need for life support. He had surrendered to the devastation forced upon himself and his family after the Gardasil injections. He was only 2 months away from turning 18 years old.

Colton's best friend played the most amazing piano piece at his funeral, performing a hit song that states how he truly walked through Hell with a smile!

Colton will always be remembered as 'Our Iron Man', while standing in the Hall of Fame, because he burns with the brightest flame!

Gardasil took Colton's physical health, his personal freedom, his precious teen years and all of his dreams for the future. Gardasil took Colton's ability to participate in life and turned him into a spectator. Modern medicine kept him alive for three precious years that we will always treasure.

He was a happy, loving, caring kid that didn't deserve the life he was given because I didn't know better. Colton's only plea was that others do their research before submitting to Gardasil injections.

He and our entire family learned the hard way - doctors are human beings – they make mistakes, just like the rest of us.

The damage Gardasil did to my son both physically and mentally is downright criminal. In an ideal world, Merck would be prosecuted for the damage they inflicted on our family. Yet they will never be held accountable for my son's life or the thousands of other lives affected by this horrific drug.

Colton's story has been shared widely and viewed by many worldwide. We want nothing more than to inform others of the true risks and side effects that can result from using Gardasil.

Please, honor Colton's memory by doing some research before you submit to HPV vaccinations.

The beginning: How all this started

By Andrea – Higganum, Connecticut USA

Korrine, nicknamed 'Korey,' was an active young lady. She enjoyed gymnastics and karate when she was younger. She took roller-skating lessons and had a real talent for this sport! Korey enjoyed her therapeutic horseback riding lessons tremendously and was quite good at it! Bicycle riding was among one of her favorite things to do!

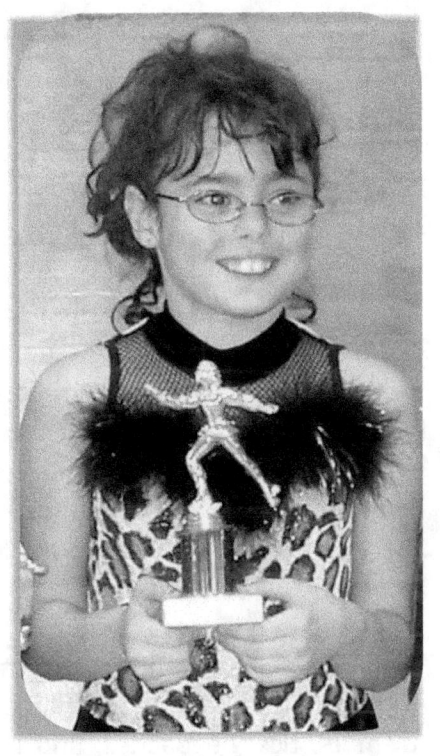

Korey was gifted with a beautiful voice. Singing was one of her hobbies, and she absolutely loved it. Music was such an important part of her life. Going to concerts was thrilling for her. She has seen Selena Gomez, Demi Lovato, Sean Mendez, and One Direction to name a few!

Korey's love of animals was so strong. She applied and was accepted to study in the Vocational Agriculture Program at Middletown High School where she achieved honor and high honors. The Program required her to earn hours volunteering in a Supervised Agriculture Experience, and Korey earned many hours working at the Ray of Light Farm on the weekends. She gave farm tours, mucked stables, led pony rides for birthday parties, and introduced the various animals to the visitors. This was such a special experience for her.

October 2, 2013 – Gardasil (HPV Vaccine) Shot #1 given with the yearly Flu Vaccine. The 2nd Gardasil Shot #2 was given on 12/3/2013. Korey never received the third and final Gardasil shot. The damage was already done and recognized by the time she was due for the final shot in the three-shot series! The first shot *seemed* uneventful, and the second shot was the beginning of a downward spiral in her physical, mental, and emotional health that has now, nearly five years later, become the living hell she and our family must cope with. Korey started to experience constant nausea and vertigo within five days of the 2nd Gardasil shot. These were the first 2 symptoms, and they were constant.

The middle: How it progressed

The first 2 symptoms of nausea and vertigo persisted and worsened over the next 6-9 months. The list of symptoms we did not understand began to grow...some subtle, some not so subtle. Korey complained of blurry vision, floaters, and sensitivity to light and the color of walls (white walls were suddenly too bright for her). She experienced a feeling as though she would pass out when standing for Concert Choir practices. We mistakenly thought this might be stage fright.

She developed separation anxiety and was not as confident, nor independent as she once was. Korey started to experience what she referred to as 'heart flutters' and a rapid beat. Her anxiety increased and she could no longer sleep in her own room. She became carsick when we traveled and would need to sit in the front seat to minimize her discomfort. Korey started to experience panic attacks often, starting in March 2014. We could not put the pieces together just yet, however, we knew that something changed and was very wrong with our daughter.

The bizarre symptom list continued to grow over the next few months: She experienced increasing fatigue, joint pain, muscle aches, tremors, tics, headaches, and neuropathy. She was not the same girl she was at the beginning of her freshman year in the VOAG Program. She could no longer participate in her Supervised Agriculture Program at Ray of Light Farm.... she could not physically muck the stalls, nor walk the farm due to her vertigo and nausea. She tried to stay on at the farm, but she did not have the stamina and always felt as though she would pass out.

The changes in Korey were difficult to process or explain. She was clearly not herself and would now cry frequently for no apparent reason. She experienced a worsening of symptoms between the spring and fall of 2014. Chest pain and tunnel vision were now added to the growing list of medical issues. She also had noticeable cognitive decline and intermittent swallowing difficulty. Korey had trouble sleeping and when she was able to fall asleep, she woke up from nightmares or hallucinations (movies playing out). The pain increased in her legs, neck, back, knees, and shoulders.

We had seen her pediatrician early on and discussed the nausea and vertigo. She offered a neurologist referral, however, we declined at this point. She referred us to a GI practice, and we did pursue this avenue. The bloodwork was all within normal ranges, and the GI could not add any answers other than chronic constipation according to Korey's health history and recent x-rays taken in the summer of 2013. The physician's assistant scheduled an exploratory colonoscopy and endoscopy which ultimately were cancelled: We opted out of this invasive procedure after a physical therapist, her vision specialist referred her to, found several muscle issues that were in the same area as her discomfort. Korey had been seeing a world renowned vision specialist, a neuro-optometrist since 2011, after experiencing some double vision. Dr. P. was able to eliminate the double vision with the use of prisms and vision therapy. He was aware of the growing list of concerns we had regarding Korey's health and referred us to a neurologist: We took him up on this recommendation and scheduled an appointment for 7/10/2014.

We waited like what seemed forever in Dr. K's waiting room, but when we got in his office, we were with him for 3 hours. He took her history, listened to her list of complaints, reviewed MRI results that were previously done due to her hearing loss (sensorineural assumed from birth), and of course, a physical exam. Initially, her presentation seemed like possible Lyme disease and/or co-infections. He touched on things we did not understand at this time: Words such as PANDAS, PANS, and more. He took 16 tubes of blood from her at this visit!!!! He modified her anxiety medication to one that he felt she would better tolerate. We made an appointment to return in one month to review the lab results.

We got a phone call from his office before our appointment to let us know Korey's vitamin D was lower than he would like, and he wanted her to supplement with vitamin D3. We met to review the lab results which were mostly normal. He discovered a genetic mutation in one of her MTHFR genes, 1 copy of a C677T mutation which we learned had to do with how her body processed folate and vitamin B12. He noted that her B12 was somewhat lower than it should be and wanted her to start on 'active' forms of B12 with folate. The MTHFR genes have to do with methylation and having the C677T mutation reduced her methylation a bit. This was not alarming at the time since her homocysteine was normal.

PANDAS was ruled out since her strep antibodies were what he deemed not a problem. However, PANS (Pediatric Acute Onset Neuro Psychiatric Syndrome) was still on the table due to the psychiatric symptoms she was experiencing. This was all very new and foreign to us, but we remained hopeful that Korey would be returned to the 'Korey' we knew and loved so much.

We followed up with Korey's neurologist, on 9/24/14 after she had a protocol of 1 intramuscular injection of Bicillin-LA for each week for five weeks. Korey had completed a mini-neuro-psychiatric test (NeuroTrax) that her neurologist gave her to complete online. We reviewed the results which showed there was something very wrong and confirmed cognitive decline. He checked and rechecked her blood pressure when standing and sitting as well as her heart rate and explained that this was the reason she felt like she would pass out when standing. The word POTS was introduced to us and another comorbidity Korey was experiencing. The mini neuropsychological test and the other clinical symptoms seemed to confirm his PANS diagnosis. He planned to see Korey next in November.

Upon our return to Korey's neurologist in November, he drew labs for The Cunningham Panel which is antibody testing that detects whether an autoimmune reaction is causing neurologic or psychiatric symptoms. This testing would support his clinical diagnosis of PANS which results from an attack on the central nervous system. He also ordered a SPECT-scan and planned to follow-up with these results at a February 2015 visit as the labs take several weeks before the results are ready. He also referred Korey to a neurologist in New York to have an EMG (Electromyography) to test muscle and nerve function.

Korey's vision seemed to be unstable: She had 3 visits to her neuro-optometrist in 2013, 2 lens changes, and 3 sessions of vision therapy. In 2014, she had 11 visits to the same neuro-optometrist resulting in 5 lens changes, and 8 vision therapy sessions.

The nurses at Korey's high school were charting her blood pressure and heart rate several times a week upon my request. One of her doctors started her on a small dose of Adderall to help with the cognitive decline.... I believe this was sometime in October of 2014. The charting of her blood pressure and heart rate revealed that the pressure would drop, and the heart rate would climb. This explained why she felt like passing out, tremendous fatigue, and weak. The Adderall was stopped before Thanksgiving since the doctor did not want this to contribute to her heart-rate issues. Korey did report that her visual symptoms would increase, and she would also see a black tunnel during these events with varying blood pressure and heart rate.

Early in December, I received a call from the school nurse. She wanted me to take Korey to the emergency room as she was very uncomfortable having her navigate the school while her blood pressure and heart rate were all over the charts. The ER staff confirmed the blood pressure and heart rate variances but reported the EKG was normal. We consulted with a cardiologist after the ER visit. Dr. Steve was my cardiologist when I was pregnant and was someone I trusted. He clearly confirmed that Korey was experiencing orthostatic hypotension and tachycardia upon standing. He ordered an echocardiogram and stress test.

We welcomed in the New Year 2015 with a SPECT-scan on January 2nd. Sadly, Korey had tremendous troubles in school from her evolving medical issues. We ultimately decided to withdraw her from the Vocational Agriculture Program she loved so much and had her return to our home district for one on one tutoring which was scheduled according to Korey's needs.

We ventured to New York in February for the EMG testing that Dr. K. requested. She also had a tilt table test there which confirmed that Korey had autonomic system dysfunction and an excessive heart rate. Her heart rate went up to 162 beats-per-minute with the head tilting and was an increase of 57 beats-per-minute from laying down face up and resting. The needle EMG testing showed an abnormal study of patchy distal demyelinating neuropathy.

We met with Korey's neurologist in February 2015 to review the molecular labs which supported his clinical diagnosis of PANS. Her Dopamine 1 Receptor (DRD1) titer was 4,000 with the normal range being 500 - 2000 and a normal mean of 1,056. Her Tubulin (TUB) was also elevated at 2,000 with the normal range being 250 – 1,000 and a normal mean of 609. Her neurologist felt these results supported his clinical diagnosis of PANS. He explained that the DRD1 results were responsible for her involuntary movements and mood disorder and the anti-Tubulin antibodies were the reason for her neuropathy. The SPECT-scan was considered normal with mild diffuse uptake in both cerebral hemispheres.

Due to these results and the EMG and tilt table testing, Dr. K. felt that IVig (intravenous immunoglobulin) would be a good treatment for her due to the neuropathy which was diagnosed as Chronic Inflammatory Demyelinating Polyneuropathy (CIDP) and autoimmune issues.

Korey started the protocol of IVig in March and continued until mid-August. This treatment was discontinued because she could no longer tolerate the headache and pain after IVig and did not feel that she was improving.

Korey started to experience an occasional seizure in February and March of 2015. The seizures became daily starting in June and continue to this day. She described what her doctor told us were 'focal', 'partial', and sadly 'grand mal' seizures. She also started to have a growing list of food allergies or reactions. She previously had no food sensitivities. However, peanut butter, blueberries, raspberries, and pineapple now gave her a tingling tongue. The list currently includes all nuts and coconut oil, gluten, soy, honey, mint, and nutmeg. Korey always had lactose-intolerant tendencies, but now she seems to be not only reactive to lactose but casein as well.

The quest to restore Korey's health sent us to many doctors. Dr. Steve, her cardiologist, referred us to a specialist in clinical cardiac electrophysiology. The echocardiogram results were normal. The stress test had confirmed what her cardiologist observed the first day he saw her.

Korey saw Dr. JK in March 2015. His impressions included the following:

- Symptoms and signs consistent with postural orthostatic tachycardia syndrome triggered by reaction to vaccine.
- Secondary neuro-pediatric anxiety/panic syndrome
- Hypermobility syndrome as continuing to #1.

He discussed lifestyle changes to help manage POTS and gave Korey a prescription to fill for two medications that are often used in POTS treatment. We opted not to try the medications at that time since she was about to start the IVig treatments. We preferred to start one protocol at a time so we know exactly what is or isn't working and what is or isn't causing adverse reactions.

August 2015 proved to be a very busy month for medical appointments. We saw a geneticist, for an Ehlers Danlos Syndrome work-up. Korey was hypermobile, and due to this and her level of pain, we wanted to rule EDS in or out. She ordered the genetic testing, and was able to rule out most of the EDS types that had genetic markers. However, hEDS (hypermobile Ehlers Danlos Syndrome) was not her specialty as it has no genetic marker. We left there with neither a yes, nor a no relative to an EDS diagnosis.

We also had an appointment with a neurologist at the same facility. One of the doctors in Korey's primary care group wanted her to be seen by another neurologist since he was not in favor of the IVig treatments. I analyzed the list of neurologists available and chose a doctor of osteopathy. Korey's primary care doctor is a DO, and we have another DO on her medical team. I thought that this would be a good choice thinking that a DO would be more integrative and open-minded. I was so very wrong!

I should have learned my lesson by this time, but in my quest to find out exactly what was wrong with Korey's health, I did not leave out any details. I felt that if I left out something, then possibly they would not be able to accurately diagnose or more important, not be able to help her regain her health. I used those two forbidden words, 'Gardasil' and 'Lyme' and I added another taboo word to the history: 'PANS'.

It is not my imagination that these words typically draw the same reaction from an "inside the box" physician, and yet again, they did with this neurologist! The result is an immediate invalidation of symptoms and causation. I usually request the physician's notes, and my thoughts are confirmed in their report. They become immediately dismissive of a serious health issue, and once again, they go to 'it's all in your head' or 'anxiety can do amazing things to your body'.

Korey's neurologist ordered a "one-hour" EEG which was pretty much useless. There were no seizures during this hour, however, the entire event prompted a panic attack. Korey felt the pressure that a one-hour test put on her. This test was a waste of our time, energy, and the insurance company's funds! We did not follow-up with this neurologist again since her attitude demonstrated exactly how not interested she was in helping Korey.

This scene would continue to play out with many of the providers we tried, but not all of them. We occasionally found an open-minded provider who was genuinely interested in Korey's medical issues, and whole-heartedly listened to her symptoms and history. These providers would agree that her case was extremely complicated and that there were several comorbidities working against her. These providers were not shocked at the thought of Gardasil injury, and they would try to help Korey.

Unfortunately, Korey was not able to be helped by many due to her body's lack of tolerance for many of the various treatments and medications. She could not tolerate even the gentlest of detoxification remedies nor could she tolerate the medications ordered for POTS or PANS or seizures without experiencing disturbing reactions.

I inquired about Korey's trying low-dose Naltrexone (LDN) since I had read extensively about this medication. Many people with autoimmune problems and many more medical issues had tremendous success with LDN. It had very few side-effects which were usually temporary and minor. We started a trial of LDN, however, Korey was so hypersensitive she could not even tolerate this medication which was compounded and made with 'clean' ingredients.

One of the therapies that helped Korey during this time was physical therapy. She was experiencing low back pain and had some success with this physical therapist. Again, Korey was extremely sensitive to touch, and many modalities we tried did not work or were too painful for her. She tried acupuncture and found that she was in a great deal of pain after the treatment. She tried other PT's and had seizures after treatment.

We had an appointment late in August 2015 with her primary care provider. He has been wonderful and has truly tried to help her wherever he could. He is not on board with a Gardasil injury so, we agreed to disagree on that issue but not dismiss it. He viewed a video of one of the grand mal seizures and was horrified by what he saw. He agreed that a one-hour EEG was a waste of time and resources and referred us to a neurologist who would conduct a three-day in hospital EEG.

As it turned out, we had a very long wait to see the neurologist and obtain the EEG. While we were waiting for these appointments, we continued pursuing the other medical issues that Korey was experiencing. Her eyesight was extremely unstable and would change between the visit to her optometrist and when new lenses were received.

Korey's primary care physician tried Midodrine to relieve Korey's POTS symptoms, and she could not tolerate the medication. He then tried Propranolol for her headaches and POTS symptoms. Again, she could not tolerate the medication. He ordered an upper GI and emptying study to evaluate Korey's constant nausea. The results were within normal limits.

The nausea continued, and the food sensitivities increased. There was a consensus from "functional" providers that she was experiencing leaky gut, so she tried several supplements for this. Korey continued her weekly visits to her therapist and monthly visits to a top-notch psychiatrist who specialized in psychopharmacology. This doctor tried many anxiety and/or depression medications, yet Korey could not tolerate any of them. If she happened to tolerate a medication, it did not help! One of the medications Korey felt was helping her prompted a very serious and potentially life-threatening rash (Steven-Johnson's) and had to be discontinued.

We paid attention to starting and trialing one medication at a time in order to be able to determine whether she could tolerate it, and if it was of any help. She tried Gabapentin with the thoughts of it possibly helping with neuropathy and seizures, however, she could not continue this drug either due to side-effects and reactions.

In January of 2016, we tried a homeopath who provided support via skype interviews that developed a comprehensive plan for detoxing the Gardasil vaccine and strengthening Korey's systems. Sadly, Korey could not even tolerate even the gentlest of liver supports and was extremely discouraged. This was very disappointing since I believed then, and still do to this date, that if Korey could get through some of this treatment she would see benefits.

We finally got in to see the new neurologist, but she turned out to be a huge disappointment through no fault of the person who referred us to her. We sat down for our initial history with her, and she focused on two of Korey's providers, her vision specialist and her neurologist. She had negative remarks about both providers which typically was rare for another provider to voice such strong, negative opinions about another professional.

As I listened to this, I remember thinking 'she was so inside the box that she could not find her way out' and that was why she was so bitter about those professionals who were both open-minded and capable of thinking outside the box.

She did order the EEG testing which was the goal. The results of the inpatient testing were what they called "Psychogenic Non-Epileptic Seizures" or PNES. They recommended Cognitive Behavior Therapy (CBT). Did we believe this diagnosis? No, we can agree that the seizures are not epileptic, however, Korey had regular CBT therapy.... this diagnosis would be too easy!

The diagnosis they gave Korey is the 'go to' diagnosis many of the Gardasil injured hear repeatedly. I interpret this to mean: 'I really don't know what is going on with your daughter,' or 'this is way too complicated for me, and I do not have the time to get to the root of the seizures'.

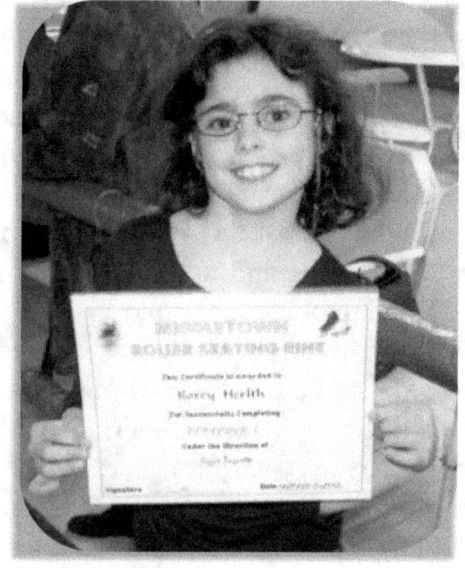

The cherry on this ice cream sundae was in her final report: She wrote that Korey was 'malingering' during her physical neurological exam and that the exam was normal!

Korey has tremors that even I can see them. Her primary neurologist has never noted a normal neurological exam for Korey. He has noted when something seemed improved or worse; In fact no neurological exam she has undergone since Gardasil has been 'normal'. Actually, 'normal' doesn't exist in our vocabulary or world since Gardasil.

I've noted 6 grand mal seizures on my calendar in March 2016. Each of these would last 30 to 45 minutes from the aura right through being unconscious and experiencing multiple convulsions. Korey tried Gabapentin, but she could not tolerate even the low doses. She also tried Keppra, Topamax, and other anti-seizure medications with no luck: They did not help, and the adverse effects were many. I believe that previously mentioned that Lamictal seemed to help the seizures, but Korey developed the early stages of the Steven-Johnson rash and had to discontinue this medication.

We tried Tai Chi lessons for our overall health and well-being. It seemed gentle enough for Korey, and she could take breaks if standing became a problem. Our schedule did not allow us to continue the Tai Chi, however, we plan to start up again when we can and reap the benefits.

Korey had a baseline Pap smear and HPV Test in April 2016. Both were thankfully negative. Of course, we had to pay out of pocket since the insurance would deny coverage for the testing no matter what the naturopath wrote! Her regular barrage of medical appointments continued as we tried to find treatments that would at least help some of her medical issues. Her vision loss continued to be unstable and progressing.

On July 12, 2016 we were on our way to a doctor's appointment when Korey told me that one of her eyelids closed! Looking at her face, we thought she may have an episode of Bell's palsy.... this was something completely new to the plethora of medical issues Korey faces daily. We made the decision to keep driving to the doctor versus going to an emergency room. Yet again, we were face to face with another 'in the box' doctor: She thought Korey was making this up....so much so that she accused her of searching for symptoms online and mimicking them!! We left shortly after *that* diagnosis and never returned to this doctor again!!

We did take a detour on the way home to chance seeing one of her team of doctors with an open-mind. A good rule of thumb that has worked for us has been to ask if the doctor was Lyme-literate. If they were, then they were not thrown off by complicated patients, even ones without Lyme or those with Lyme plus comorbidities. We were fortunate to find such a physician's assistant. He gave Korey a shot of B12 as this helped another of his patients in the past with this problem. He told us not to let this go if it did not improve within 24 hours and to see her visual specialist the very next day.

When Korey woke up the next day, both eyelids were closed. We called and went to see her vision specialist who thought allergies might be the root of the ptosis (technical term for what was happening) and suggested Korey try Benadryl and return in a few days for follow-up. He also called Korey's (Team Korey) neurologist to discuss the ptosis before we left the office. Her neurologist wanted to have us see him the very next day. We took the trip to see Dr. K. who felt that this was possibly Myasthenia Gravis which warranted an ER trip and MRI with further testing of labs, etc... The labs came back negative, however, there is a 50% chance that they would be negative, and the MRI series of tests came back normal. This did not rule out MG in his eyes: He started Korey on a trial of Mestinon (Pyridostigmine) which is the medication for Myasthenia Gravis. Unfortunately, she could not tolerate the medication and needed to stop it. The ptosis improved

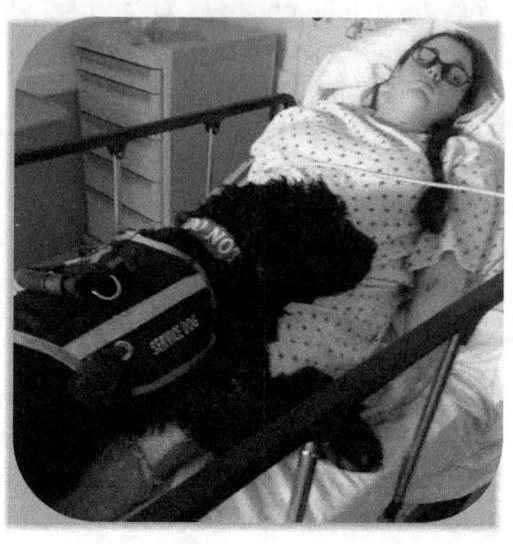

some, however she still battles this intermittently to this day. All of us keep this in mind going forward. I feel it necessary to point out that 3 of her regular Team Korey doctors did not even remotely think that she was fabricating the ptosis!

On July 27th, (2016) Korey went to Danbury Hospital for a follow-up SPECT-scan (previous SPECT done on January 2, 2015) which was ordered by Dr. K. to see how Korey's brain was functioning. As we understand his explanation, the MRI shows the parts of the brain and lesions, if any; the SPECT-scan shows the function of the brain and blood flow.

While waiting for the results of the SPECT-scan, we had appointments with a neuro-ophthalmologist to pursue the MG issue.... what an experience for the books! The doctor was pregnant, and I can only hope her rude bedside manner was due to hormones. Her behavior should not be dismissed even for that explanation. Once again, we were met with political agenda and prejudice....it was obvious that this doctor and the senior partner in the group were not fans of the neuro-optometrist Korey has been with since 2011. I guess the medical politics of neuro-ophthalmologist vs. neuro-optometrist sometimes overshadows what is best for the patient. We sought out the ophthalmologist because MG is a medical diagnosis, so the manual MG tests could be done at this practice.

There were 2 tests performed specific to Myasthenia Gravis, an ice test and a sleep test. Both tests were *POSITIVE*. In spite of the results, this doctor said she was not *'giving'* Korey the MG diagnosis and that anxiety could do funny things to a person.

At this point, I thoughtfully asked her how frequent she would see Korey if she were to become her patient, and her response sealed all the above, *'once a year'*. She felt that Korey, a person with unstable and progressive vision loss and multiple lens changes within a year would only need to be followed once a year!! Really?!!! You just cannot make this stuff up!

Dr. K. gave us a referral to a medical marijuana doctor so that Korey could participate in the legal CT MMJ Program. We saw the doctor, got the paperwork, and finally with our cards in hand went to the dispensary. We made several trips back and forth to the dispensary, but for some reason, the pharmacist insisted that she was giving us the correct products based on Korey's symptoms, but they were not working for Korey!

On September 8, 2016, we ventured to Long Island for several stand-up MRI tests ordered by the chiropractor that the vision specialist referred Korey to for her neck issues. He had patients that improved quite a bit under this doctor's care. The results were interesting and showed soft tissue issues which might have to do with findings relative to C1/C2 rotation, disc bulges in two areas of her cervical spine, and decreased cervical spinal fluid flow in both caudocranial and craniocaudal directions.

We finally met with the neurologist to review the SPECT-scan results. There was a change from the first one in January to the 2nd one in July. There was reduced blood flow in the cerebral cortex as well as other areas of Korey's brain. Dr. K felt this supported his official diagnoses of:

- Post Vaccination Autoimmune Encephalopathy
- Post Vaccination Autoimmune Autonomic Dysfunction
- Post Vaccination Autoimmune Peripheral Neuropathy
- Potentially Post Vaccination Autoimmune Vasculitis

All these and what the neurologist who did the nerve conduction testing diagnosed as CIDP (Chronic Inflammatory Demyelinating Polyneuropathy. Dr. K. encouraged Korey to try IVIG again and she agreed.

IVIG started on October 17, 2016: A homecare IV nurse, would travel from Rhode Island driving 1 ½ hours to our house and give Korey the pre-medications and IVIG infusion which would take approximately 10 – 11 hours. If they tried to run the infusion any faster, Korey's side-effects would escalate. The plan was that Korey would have IVIG infusions every other week.

In January 2017, her vision specialist referred Korey to a doctor of osteopathy, for osteopathic manipulation to help with her vision and also overall health and well-being. Dr. T. has been a keeper and a member of Team Korey. He is Lyme-literate and a doctor of the complicated patient. He does not get discouraged easily and is capable of thinking outside the box. This medical practice was not entirely new for us. The doctor of osteopathy referred Korey to Dr. J. (his wife) in 2012 to help with an ankle injury. This is one of my favorite Practices since being doctors of osteopathy, they could provide mainstream medical care and also offer integrative care as well with alternatives to antibiotics, etc. while seeking the root of the illness. They were able to give Korey the saline IV's when her POTS flared and do so in a fraction of the time we would spend in the emergency room at a fraction of the ER cost!

February 2017 - we had an appointment with a pulmonologist for her asthma and breathing issues. Korey had seen her primary care physician for trouble breathing in the past and had the standard spirometry testing. The results were not great. It was thought that her asthma was flaring. This was strange since Korey had moderate asthma as a child, but it was very well controlled and had tapered off as she grew older. She had been off asthma medications for quite a while now.

Is it possible that her asthma has returned? I suppose so, however, Korey insisted that this feeling was different. Korey went for a full battery of pulmonary function testing which showed that the cause of her breathing issues was indeed asthma. She started up with her full asthma plan of Singulair and Flovent daily and her rescue inhaler when needed.

In between all the medical appointments, Korey tried to continue her education with her one on one tutor completing assignments and earn hours needed for Transition Class by volunteering in the local library to cut out relevant articles from the newspaper for their scrapbook. Unfortunately she had to decline this opportunity to earn transition hours due to her progressive vision loss. The newsprint was pretty small, and the CCTV Magnifier was just too cumbersome for this assignment. She was able to assist in the main office of her high school to gain the necessary transition hours by sorting and distributing mail and working on any projects they had for her.

She continued to be followed-up by the cardiologist, at least twice a year for an echocardiogram and follow-up appointment regarding her POTS. We visited Massachusetts Eye and Ear on May 15, 2017 regarding Korey's vision. I am not sure that they had us in the appropriate specialty. Nevertheless, Korey endured the entire day of testing. We met with the retina specialist at the end of the day, and he said everything looked fine and wished her well.

This was discouraging news as we truly hoped for a complete understanding of Korey's vision loss. At least he was a gentleman and not rude. We have seen and experienced rude many times during this journey!

June was very busy for us as Korey had required interviews to complete for Transition, IVIG, meetings for a State Program for 30 hours of employment in the summer, as well as preparing for Senior Prom and Graduation. Yes, Graduation!

She did it with the help of her very committed tutor, Lori, who would read to Korey when she could not see, who would write for her when she was too tired to write. They did it!

Oh, and of course, Max, Korey's guide and service dog accompanied her and a friend to the Prom, and he even walked with Korey for Graduation. She walked for graduation and received a certificate of attendance, but she needed to return in the fall to complete a few more requirements for the final diploma. To be able to walk with her class was thrilling for her and us!

July found us continuing the quest to find just the right provider and just the right protocol to help Korey. We tried an appointment with an endocrinologist who was highly recommended. Once he looked over her history, he gave the okay to his staff to make an appointment for her. They sent us a lab slip and had bloodwork done prior to the appointment which was a good timesaver. The labs included some we had never run before, and they were all in the normal ranges. He sold us some supplements and then there was no further follow-up on his end. Korey and I agreed that he was very close to retiring and that his steam to deal with complicated cases had dwindled. This was not a person to include on her care team.

Korey's 30-hour placement for the Transition Level-up Program was with a Credit Union for a Union very close to our home. She attended a

5-hour orientation for the Level-Up Program which included completing the necessary work paperwork such as tax forms, etc...

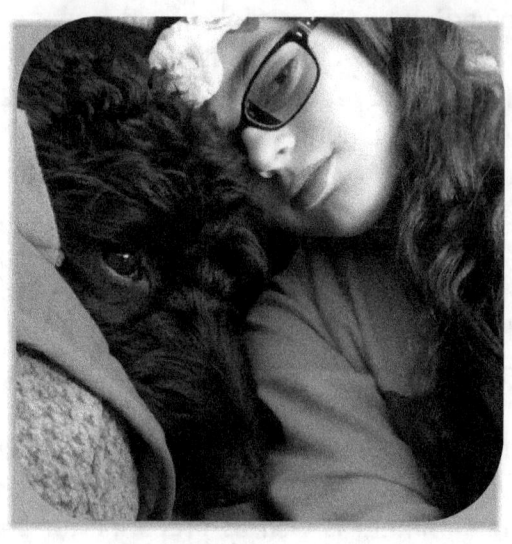

We also had an appointment with a neuro-ophthalmologist at a leading teaching hospital in New Haven, Connecticut. Korey's vision specialist, had referred her to this individual in an effort to identify the cause of her vision instability and loss. The doctor reviewed the information from our visit to Massachusetts Eye and Ear as well as the other neuro-ophthalmologist we saw in 2016 after the Ptosis episode and the visit summaries from Dr. P. Once again, Korey was basically discounted. This doctor was polite, but her notes documented how much time she personally spent with us and without offering any findings.

Korey completed her 30-hour work with the Level-Up Program through The State of Connecticut. Her work program was set-up to work around her being chronically ill and having many appointments. She matched up invoices and filed for the employer. It was difficult with her vision issues, however, she was determined and plugged along. Working in addition to all she faced daily was a huge drain, but Korey so wanted to have some semblance of a 'normal' life.

Her primary neurologist switched Korey to subcutaneous IG infusions in September. The intravenous IG was so draining on her, and the side-effects were the same as when she started. The IVIG would take 10 – 11 hours to run to keep the side-effects to a minimum. My husband, John, and I learned how to give her the subcutaneous IG and started this process in September 2017.

We saw her vision specialist, neuro-optometrist, several times in September and reviewed the results from our visit to a neuro-ophthalmologist at a leading teaching Hospital in New Haven, CT. He referred us to a leading hospital eye center in Baltimore, and we had an appointment on October 3rd. This appointment was life-changing for

Korey. She was finally able to get validation from a renowned physician AND a piece of the complicated puzzle uncovered. We were so very fortunate that he was very well-versed in Ehlers-Danlos and knew the questions to ask as he reviewed her history. Even more than that, he truly listened to what she had to say. His response to her was "You are no pretty little liar, I believe you have Ehlers-Danlos Syndrome". EDS is a connective tissue syndrome, and this explained a great deal of Korey's pain and joint popping.

Dr. S. referred Korey to a leading EDS geneticist in Baltimore. He emailed her while we were there! Dr. S. was different than all the previous eye specialists that saw Korey. He did not think she was malingering or exaggerating or seeking attention. He did not find the cause of her vision loss or instability; however, he did not question whether this was 'not real'. This exam deemed her legally blind.

Korey finally had validation that she knew more about her body than many of the professionals she had seen over the past 4 years. Her regular vision specialist, her neurologist, her doctor of osteopathy, and her primary care doctor always knew she was reporting exactly what was happening to her, and now she had an objective doctor solve a huge piece of her complicated puzzle. Best of all, he did not call her symptoms 'a psychiatric problem'.

Life was and remains very busy in the quest to uncover how to heal Korey. The very next week she was due to have a sleep study. She had been complaining of waking up in the middle of the night and gasping for her breath. She had been having a great deal of sleep or lack of sleep troubles since Gardasil and now was experiencing day and night time breathing issues. Korey's primary neurologist had ordered the sleep study. The results further validated Korey's knowledge of her body and that she tells the truth. She had mild sleep apnea and hypoxia! It was recommended that Korey start using a CPAP machine for her sleep apnea and hypoxia at night. She continued seeing the pulmonologist to try and resolve her breathing issues during the day.

I know that I stress validation as being huge. The Gardasil-injured have spent so much time, energy, and money trying to find the protocol(s) that would successfully heal them only to be labeled as malingering, psychologically unstable, conversion disorder, and attention seekers.

Their families, usually the moms, are thought and some have been outright accused of having Munchausen by Proxy Syndrome which is a mental illness where a caregiver fabricates illness and symptoms. It is a form of child abuse!

The invalidation and repeated disrespect from medical providers are very damaging to the injured and their families. Gardasil injury evolves....it is not just one symptom, or one syndrome or disease. It is extremely complicated and presents in most with many comorbidities, and it is most certainly REAL.

Our family ended 2017 with more pieces of the puzzle in place and better informed about just how damaging Gardasil injury is to a person, especially someone who might be predisposed or susceptible to such an injury.

From what we know today, Gardasil cannot cause hEDS, it is hereditary. However, as in Korey's case, her hEDS was not front and center.... she had subtle signs and markers of it, but she was not living hEDS. Gardasil triggered her hEDS to activate and advance and add quite a bit to her medical plate which was already full.

We entered 2018 hopeful that we might provide Korey with more answers and some healing of what has become an enormous mound of different syndromes. This is not Munchausen: This is the life of a Gardasil injured person and family.... a living hell.

We were very fortunate to get an appointment on the books to see the geneticist we were referred to by Dr. S (Baltimore) for February 2nd, 2018. While we anxiously waited for the appointment, I was looking for a comprehensive physical therapy program for Korey and was referred to a wonderful facility: The Hospital for Special Care in New Britain, Connecticut. They have an incredible outpatient program which includes aqua and land physical therapy.

Korey did very well with the aqua therapy in the 'cooler' of the two pools. There is a heated pool which serves some people very well but was tough on her POTS. She started treatment at this facility in January of 2018 and has had some occupational therapy here as well. The staff are very knowledgeable of EDS, and Korey's physical therapy was phenomenal. Tricia was able to get Korey to wear a supportive sneaker which is critical for someone with hypermobile EDS....this is the first pair of sneakers we purchased that Korey wears nearly every day!

BESB (Board of Education Services for the Blind) set up an appointment for Korey to be evaluated by a low-vision specialist, Dr. RK. We saw Dr. RK, and he felt that Korey's vision loss was beyond the assisted technology level of a CCTV (Closed Circuit TV Magnifier) and that she needed text to speech technology. He knew Korey's neuro-optometrist, and said she was seeing the best. Dr. RK's evaluation confirmed that Korey was now *legally blind*.

How could this be? Dr. P. had improved her vision with prisms, and she was quite stable in his care from 2011 through most of 2013. Truly, it was after the 2nd Gardasil shot that she reported blurry vision and floaters. Her vision seemed to progressively become unstable and finally deteriorated to being legally blind.

February 2nd finally came, and we traveled to Baltimore to see Dr. F. who is a renowned EDS Specialist. Finally, a great deal of validation of Korey's physical complaints. I am not sure why other providers (2 neurologists and 3 neuro-ophthalmologists) noted normal neurological exams. The results of this physical exam neurologically and otherwise were anything but normal! We left the office with a 13-page summary of the visit and findings.

The diagnoses included POTS, MCAS or MCAD (Mast Cell Activation Syndrome /Disorder), and a connective tissue disorder, most likely hypermobile Ehlers-Danlos Syndrome (hEDS). Dr. F. ran a panel of genetic tests since there are currently 14 types of EDS: hEDS has not been linked to a gene to date. We headed for home with the 13-page report filled with not only history and physical exam information but also with recommendations and orders from the doctor for several tests, medications, and specialists to see. Dr. F. wanted Korey to be seen by a pain specialist, a urologist for urodynamic testing to rule out tethered cord, and to have specific radiological testing done. Our discussion with Dr. F. did not include Gardasil. It was noted in her history, however, we stressed to her that we were there to confirm Korey had Ehlers-Danlos and were not looking for her to pursue a Gardasil injury. I was afraid she would not accept Korey as a patient.... she did not have to since her wait list was currently three years out.

We followed up on the testing recommendation for a specific CT-scan to rule out CCI (Cranio-Cervical Instability). It turned out 3 different CT-scans were required, and the facility would only do one noting that it was just too much radiation to do more than one at a time. The result was that cranio-cervical instability could not be ruled out or confirmed as a problem.

We traveled to Rhode Island to see a urologist, Dr. S. who conducted a Cystometrogram, and we drove to New York for the stand-up MRI's that she requested. Connecticut does not have any stand-up MRI facilities! The Cystometrogram was repeated twice and not the most comfortable test either. Again, it did not rule out tethered cord or confirm it. It did show that Korey had some bladder dysfunction which is not surprising since autonomic nervous system failure includes bladder issues. The stand-up MRI's showed pretty much the same findings as the previous set of tests in September 2016.

February also came with the usual doctor appointments and testing. The pulmonologist ordered more breathing tests to get to the bottom of her random shortness of breath and dropping oxygen saturations. The results were not normal, but the doctor was at a loss to explain this other than noting asthma had worsened.

We completed the last of the EDS geneticist's recommendations in April and had an appointment with a knowledgeable pain specialist. Due to Korey's hypersensitivity to medications, the pain specialist recommended trying a low and slow (low-dose and slow increase) pain patch, Butrans.

Korey was a trooper and stuck with this through several dose increases, however, she could not tolerate this medication and only received minimal relief. The next trial was for low-dose Naltrexone (LDN). This would be Korey's third trial with LDN. LDN has helped many of the Gardasil injured and those with autoimmune issues. She gave this a good try, but after the dose increase, she experienced side-effects once again and had to discontinue the LDN.

In May we tried yet another neuro-ophthalmologist that was highly recommended by my eye doctor. This specialist was her go-to for the complicated eye issues. He agreed to see Korey and once again we were cautiously optimistic that we might get some answers for the reason she was legally blind now and had hardly any peripheral vision. This visit tied a previous emergency room visit for the absolute rudest provider yet. After several tests, he asked Korey, "Why are you here?" and she responded, "I want to know why I am losing my vision". His response was "There is nothing wrong with your eyes. This is a psychiatric problem, and you need to see a psychiatrist".

This broke her beyond belief. We took our medical records and left. We happened to stop at Korey's neurologist prior to going home as I needed to drop something there. I met Dr. K. in the hall, and he asked where Korey was…. I told him what just happened and that she was in the car crying. He was so upset and said to make an appointment with him so that he could support her. He agreed with me that the psychiatric diagnosis would be too easy. This was not a mental health issue: The vision did not come and go, it progressed and involved central vision and peripheral vision.

In June, I presented a doctor of osteopathy with supporting documentation as to why I wanted to run some specific POTS testing on Korey. He agreed and ordered and drew the labs which needed to be sent to Germany. CellTrend in Germany was the only lab to run a POTS Panel which could detect certain autoantibodies that some of the Gardasil injured were coming up positive with and we hoped this would lead us to a treatment direction if she were positive for some of the autoantibodies.

This testing was not a waste of the over $500 we paid out of pocket nor of all the efforts to get her blood sent to Germany. She had two of the antibodies return 'at risk' (AT1R and ETAR) and was positive for two anti-adrenergic antibodies (Anti a-1 and Anti b-2P), two of the adrenergic antibodies were negative (a-2 and b-1). She was also positive for three of the anti-Muscarinic Cholinergic Receptor Antibodies (Receptor 1, Receptor 3, and Receptor 4) and negative for two of this type of antibodies (Receptor 2 and Receptor 5). This was obviously more medically technical than we could understand, however, it meant a great deal to Dr. K. and Dr. T. in that Korey had all these antibodies that she should not have had pointing to an autoimmune origin and more than likely the cause of her Gardasil injury or part of it if we are being conservative. Dr. K. also felt this explained some of the ptosis and Myasthenia Gravis symptoms. The CellTrend testing and results was another huge piece of the puzzle solved.

Dr. K. felt that Korey needed IVIG treatment again but this time, she needed Rituximab (Rituxan) which was a very powerful drug used in cancer treatments to kill cells. The hope was that this medication would kill the autoantibodies that she should not have and that the IVIG would replenish her immune system. He ran the preliminary labs to make sure she was stable enough to receive such a rigorous treatment. One test he explained to us was for something called the JC Virus antibodies (John Cunningham) which screened blood to see if a person could or could not have Rituximab. We researched the JC Virus antibodies while awaiting the lab results. The JC virus is common and dormant in about 80% of the public, however, if the antibodies are too high, Rituximab cannot be considered as a safe treatment. Korey's lab results returned with a very high JC virus result of 3.43 (the low positive was 0.40)! Dr. K. told us that she could not have the Rituximab treatment since she was at a high risk for a complication of PML (Progressive multifocal leukoencephalopathy) due to the medication, and PML is fatal. PML is a demyelinating brain infection due to the JC Virus. This news was devastating!

Dr. K. was also pursuing a referral to a lost vision specialist at Massachusetts Eye and Ear. Korey had researched and found information on this doctor there who specialized in unknown lost vision cases. Dr. P. felt this was a good idea since her last OCT (Optical Coherence Tomography) test pointed to cortical blindness and the possibility that reduced cerebral perfusion might be responsible for Korey's vision loss. An OCT is a light wave test and non-invasive which takes cross-section pictures of the retina. Dr. T. called this specialist about Korey's vision and is working on the documentation needed to prioritize an appointment with Dr. R. at MA Eye and Ear. He did agree to see Korey! Time seems to stand still when you are awaiting appointment scheduling and for the appointments themselves!

Korey had her wisdom teeth removed in August! This was no routine matter for someone with a MTHFR mutation, hypermobile Ehlers-Danlos, and POTS! Oh, we cannot forget asthma either! Her oral surgeon was wonderful and cautious. There was no way he was going to attempt this surgery in the office. He contacted the head of anesthesia at the hospital that he was affiliated with, and they decided it was in Korey's best interest to have the surgery at the main campus at the hospital itself. Dr. C. and this hospital were totally on their game, and the surgery went very well without any complications. Korey seemed to heal well as we held our breath at each follow-up visit until one day she had terrible pain in her lower cheek.... Dr. C. confirmed this was an infection and prescribed a course of antibiotics. He also confirmed that Korey's jaw was dislocated due to her connective tissue syndrome, hEDS! This took quite a while to clear up, and to date her jaw is closer to being back in place but not 100% there. Korey is a trooper as the pain was intense.

She had another surprise in lab results. She was positive for Babesia Microti which is a Lyme-associated and tick-borne disease of a specific parasite in the red blood cells. Thank God for Dr. K. being Lyme-literate.... we did not even know he tested her for Lyme when the labs were drawn. She is currently on a course of anti-malaria antibiotics for the Babesia Microti. Once again, Korey is a real trooper and tries hard to tolerate the gastrointestinal side-effects from the medication.

In following up with Korey's pain doctor, we decided to try Ketamine infusions for her pain. We had tried these once before with a psychiatrist that tried many medications for Korey's PANS symptoms which included anxiety and depression. The Ketamine infusions were the latest and greatest hope for medication resistant depression. This was two years ago and infused via a different protocol. Dr. C. said he would go low and slow with this knowing that Korey is hypersensitive to medications. He also planned to give her nausea medication and a relaxing medication to help avoid any hallucinations during the infusion. Dr. C. is an anesthesiologist and has worked with Ketamine for many years. Korey feels very reassured by this and is currently going to receive her 6th infusion next week. So far, she has tolerated a dose increase and feels a bit of a subtle but not long-lasting improvement in her pain.

She did have a seizure during one infusion when it ran a bit faster than anticipated. Dr. C. swiftly gave her some Versed which stopped the seizure. The following infusion ran extremely slow and next week he anticipates a small increase in dose but extending the infusion over 3 ½ hours to reduce her side effects. We hope that this protocol will give her some lasting relief of pain and at the same time take the edge off her depression and anxiety.

Dr. C. recommended we visit the marijuana dispensary and add a CBD (Cannabidiol) vape to her protocol for seizures. We made an appointment and picked up the CBD last week.

As you can see, November has proved to be another busy 'medical' month. Korey had her follow-up echocardiogram two weeks ago which was normal. Dr. Steve, her cardiologist, feels it is important to have an echocardiogram twice a year due to her hEDS, and he will see her in January 2019 to review her POTS and hEDS status. We will also provide him with the CellTrend antibody results as they do have cardiac implications.

Korey asked me to set up a gynecologist appointment for her as she has been experiencing severe lower abdominal discomfort (pain). I contacted my doctor's office to make the appointment and requested an HPV test and Pap smear be done for her. The receptionist told me that they would not do this for someone under 21, and I informed her that Korey was Gardasil injured and had a baseline of both tests before,

I intended to pay for this knowing that insurance would not pay for someone under 21, and this was necessary follow-up to being Gardasil injured. She made the appointment. I did not accompany Korey on this appointment, and her doctor refused to do the requested testing saying it was not necessary!

Once again, the mention of the words Gardasil injured and the mainstream medical response of denial by asserting the power of not testing as requested. I am livid at the bold disrespect of this provider. We will get the testing done somewhere else, but Korey must go through the entire internal exam again which is not pleasant. The

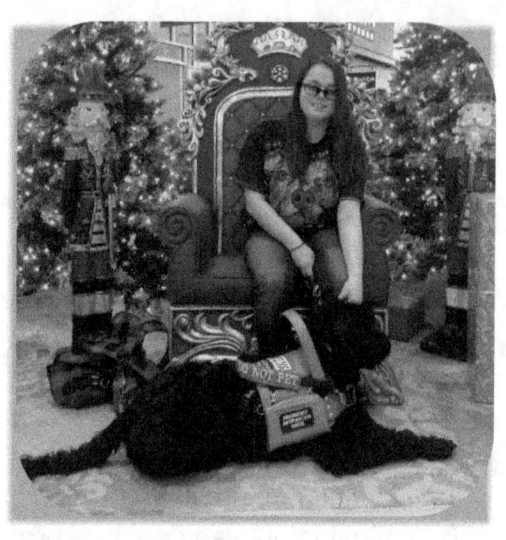

doctor did say that Korey was experiencing some pelvic floor dysfunction and recommended exercises to resolve this.

Today is Saturday, December 1st, 2018, and Monday, December 3rd will be the 5th anniversary of the fateful 2nd booster of Gardasil that changed Korey's life and ours. I would be remiss if I did not introduce Max to you. Max is Korey's Labradoodle who provides her with guide and service dog assistance so that Korey could be as independent as possible and feel safe in public and at home.

When medications did not help or could not be tolerated, Max, Korey's Labradoodle stepped up to the plate….

As Korey's health continued to decline, and she was on homebound studies, she became afraid to leave our home; home was her safe place. She started to work with her dog, Max, a black Labradoodle, and our other two dogs, Bruno and Ollie.

At first, she was teaching them basic dog behavior, but soon she realized Max's potential to be a service dog! When Korey was a student in the VOAG Program, her area of interest was in becoming a service dog trainer. She had done and continued to pursue researching service dog training. Korey started to work with Max specifically to train him on service dog tasks that would help her be more independent such as item retrieval, deep pressure therapy, some light mobility for POTS symptoms, and more.

Max was a natural when the seizures started in 2015; he instinctively could detect by smell whatever chemical she gave off, and that behavior was shaped; he would alert her by whining and or licking her face, and he would alert us by barking. He was able to alert to a pending seizure about 10 to 30 minutes before it started so that she could get herself to a safe spot on the floor. At first, my husband and I did not quite 'get' what he was telling us.... we thought he wanted to go outside, however, he would refuse. Fortunately, we figured out that he was frantically telling us that Korey needed assistance. Once the seizure would start, he would lay down and give her light but still deep pressure therapy. Deep pressure therapy is a task he learned to help her manage panic attacks and other PANS symptoms.

Max was successful in assisting Korey in her time of need. Eventually, she was willing to try going out to the grocery store with Max and me for a short trip. The short trip expanded to a small shopping mall to buy clothing, and there was no doubt that Korey and Max were a great team! The locations we chose to visit were well-suited to a chronically ill person as there were benches and seating readily available. She and Max would take breaks as needed if he alerted to her tachycardia by nudging her repeatedly, and the malls offered a nice opportunity for sitting and taking a break when needed.

These 'field trips' paved the way for Korey to be able to go out to a restaurant. Max was better behaved than most of the people! She received many compliments on Max. Sometimes people would engage in discussing service dogs and tasks with her. These trips proved critical to Korey being able to lead a somewhat 'normal' life. Eventually, she was confident enough to venture out with Max and a friend or two knowing that he would keep her safe.

Some NOT so fun Facts:

Since that fateful year 2013 when Korey had her two shots of the HPV vaccine she has had 22 emergency room visits as serious health problems arose, and which required immediate medical attention. Prior to 2013, and over 15 years our girl only had to visit the ER twice. That is the difference between normal living and living with a toxic vaccine in your body which in our Korey's case has got out of control. This has also been shown to be the case in the number of specialist doctors/practitioners we have had to take Korey to in our desperate need to get someone to help our daughter and make her well.

As you have read, Korey's body appears to have reacted so badly to Gardasil that it reacts also to any treatments being given to try and counteract the damage that has been done.

Over the five years since vaccination we have visited approximately 55 different specialists from neurologists to cardiologists to speech therapists to visual experts – we have been around the circuit as you would say and yet my lovely daughter is still very ill.

I would desperately like to believe that we would not need to go back to the ER or visit another specialist doctor but that will not be the case. We pray and hope that there is someone out there who will say to us "I know how to help Korey".

That is our dream.

The End?

Will there ever be an end to the damage that Gardasil has inflicted on Korey? December 3, 2018 will be 5 years since Korey received the 2nd Gardasil shot that seemed to put her over the edge to a cascading storm of adverse reactions. There does not seem to be an end in sight to the damage, adverse reactions, and injury that Gardasil has brought to Korey and to us. Our lives have been forever changed over the past nearly five years…. physically, emotionally, socially, and financially.

I have said it before, and it still is true: ***If I could turn back time, Korey would never ever have received the HPV Vaccine, Gardasil.***

She would still be able to roller-skate, ride a horse, and enjoy a stroll on her bike. We would still enjoy time away at Rocking Horse Ranch in New York where she would enjoy the rock-climbing wall and bungee activities. She would have continued in the Vocational Agriculture Program she loved so much. There was so much she had to look forward to in life.

The cold reality as I write this is that she is now 20-years-old. She cannot drive due to seizures, cognitive decline, and loss of vision. Korey is legally blind. We have not found the root cause of the vision issues yet, however, we continue to seek more answers.

Our lives seem to be consumed with the words POTS, PANS, Post Vaccination Autoimmune Encephalopathy, Neuropathy, Raynaud's, Ptosis, leaky gut, and Mast Cell Activation Syndrome, hereditary connective tissue disorder (hEDS) or hypermobile Ehlers Danlos Syndrome and autoimmune antibodies that she should not have.

We have solved some pieces of the puzzle, however, each time we unravel one health issue, there seems to be two more that unfold.

Two things I ask of anyone reading this:

Please keep Korey in your prayers, and please do not give your child the HPV Vaccine. The latest research paper I read a few days ago supports Gardasil injury by a susceptible population and vaccinating with Gardasil at this point is the equivalent to playing roulette with your child's life…. My opinion, but this is exactly what happened to Korey.

I am hoping that the response to the research paper will be to conduct true studies with true placebos. I am in the process of reading a recently released book with respect to HPV science, *The HPV Vaccine on Trial – Seeking Justice for a Generation Betrayed,* by Mary Holland, J.D. Kim Mack Rosenberg, J.D., and Eileen Iorio. I have been sickened at the workings of Gardasil's manufacturer, Merck and the FDA and CDC among other agencies.

Cattle going to slaughter have been treated with more compassion and respect than the children given the Gardasil vaccine. The science and injustices are well-documented, and even though I thought I was well-versed in the fast-tracking of Gardasil, I could not have imagined what I am reading in this book.

The last three thoughts I would like to share with you are the following:

SaneVax (www.sanevax.org) has been my lifeline these past few years. I happened to read a story on Facebook about a young girl from Pennsylvania…This story entitled, *The Decision We Will Always Regret*, rang so familiar to me that I could not forget it. The story was published on SaneVax's website, and I reached out to them to put me in contact with the mom who wrote it. The rest is history! I owe a huge debt of gratitude to Kim and Katie for their story awakening me to what happened to Korey. I also would be remiss to not mention Norma Erickson and Freda Birrell for their hard work and dedication to all the Gardasil injured and their families…. they are working to prevent future injuries to unsuspecting people. Freda has been my lifeline, and the other moms and dads of the Gardasil injured have become my 'Gardahell' family.

We are forever grateful to Dr. P…, Dr. K…, Dr. M…, and Dr. B… for never giving up on Korey and for knowing that 'this is real'.

Vaccine Court or VICP (Vaccine Injury Compensation Program): I have not broached this subject in my writing. I have much to say on this process, however, we do have a case pending as of this writing. I will have to save my experience with the VICP for another day and another writing. Thanks to Kim, Katie, the SaneVax team, and the timeline of symptoms we compiled, we were able to piece together the connection between Korey's medical downward spiral and the 2nd dose of Gardasil, and we were able to put this together within the limits to file a claim.

Canada

Canada approved Gardasil for use in June of 2006 for females ages 9 through 26. In 2010 Gardasil was also approved for males of the same age group. The same year, Cervarix gained approval for females. As additional information came in, Canada adjusted their recommendations. This happened in 2012, 2015, 2016 and 2017. In 2015, Gardasil 9 received marketing approval. In October 2018, the recommended ages for HPV vaccine administration were extended to include both males and females through age 45. It is interesting to note Cervarix was not approved for use in the male population.[22] Currently, all three HPV vaccines are available in Canada.

In 2013, The Public Health Agency of Canada (PHAC) asked Statistics Canada to conduct a National Immunization Coverage Survey. The results showed that nearly 75% of Canadian girls age 12 to 16 had utilized HPV vaccines.[23] One year later, the 2014 adult National Immunization Coverage Survey showed 44.7% of the population ages 18 to 26, both male and female, had at least one injection of HPV vaccine. Only 8.3% of Canadian women age 27 through 45 had received at least one injection.[24]

Children between the ages of 14 and 17 are allowed to make their own medical decisions in Canada as long as the proposed treatment is necessary for their health.[25] This means any child can consent to HPV

---

[22] Public Health Services Canada; Human Papillomavirus (HPV) Prevention and HPV Vaccines: Questions and Answers; modified 2017-20-04; accessed March 2019

[23] Public Health Services Canada; Vaccine coverage in Canadian children: Highlights from the 2013 childhood National Immunization Coverage Survey (cNICS); modified 2016-10-13; accessed March 2019

[24] Public Health Services Canada; Vaccine uptake in Canadian adults: results from the 2014 adult National Immunization Coverage Survey; modified 2016-02-24; accessed March 2019

[25] Staff writer; Medical Decisions for Children 14 to 17 Years Old; educaloi.qc.ca; accessed March 2019

vaccinations whether they are administered in a school, or medical setting.

Catastrophic Loss

By Linda Morin, Quebec, Canada

I'm writing these lines to honor the memory of my lovely daughter Annabelle, who passed at 14 years old, only 15 days after receiving her second shot of HPV vaccine Gardasil.

This is our story

Annabelle was born on December 26, 1993. At the time, I was single, 34 years old and living with my father. Annabelle was the first grand-daughter and the first niece to be born in our family. We all said at the time, *she was a gift from God.* From the moment she was born, Annabelle was surrounded with a lot of love from my parents and all of my siblings.

The moment I saw her my life changed. When I looked at her, tears would roll down my cheeks. I loved her so much that my heart hurt.

During the time I was pregnant, I lived with my father and his wife (my best friend) Ginette. Needless to say, we were all really close and they were quite attached to Annabelle. Annabelle and I lived with them for the first 15 months of her life.

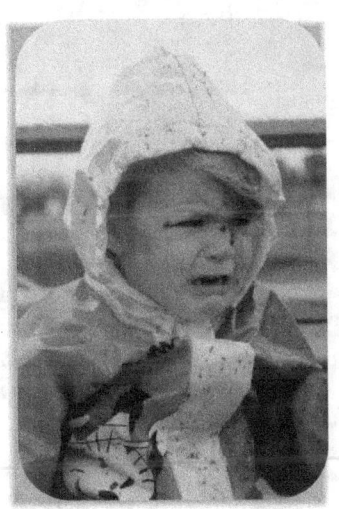

My father was a race horse breeder and trainer. He even named one of his horses, Annabelle Mor, after my precious daughter.

At a very young age, Dad would hold Annabelle in his arms during practice runs on the race track. She loved it so much she could never get enough. I remember one day it was raining and there was a lot of mud on the track. After one lap, Annabelle was full of mud on her pretty face and all over. We had to take her off the sulky. She cried so much, she cried the whole practice and kept begging her grandfather to take her back. I couldn't resist taking the time to get this memorable picture.

With every passing year, she was getting closer to her grandfather. They had the same passion: horses. I could honestly say they became best friends. Annabelle stayed at the farm every other weekend, helping out and working with her mentor because that's who he was for her. They had developed a special bond. During a regular week they would talk a few times, always about horses.

When Annabelle was eighteen months old, I met Michel. He was divorced and the father of Pier-Luc, 6-years-old, and Karine, 16-years-old. After only a week, I knew I would marry him one day.

After 2 years of being a couple, we bought a house together and decided I was going to be a stay at home Mom full time for the kids. We had become a family. Our house was near the school so the kids could walk and come home for lunch. Life was perfect. We were all very happy.

As a young girl, Annabelle was always very responsible. We could talk about anything. Our relationship was based on mutual respect and honesty. I used to always explain everything to her. We had no secrets, except about her biological father. One day, I made a promise to her that at the age of eighteen I would give her all the information about him.

Through the years, she was a volunteer at the SPCA. She went door-to-door, getting signatures to pass a law to protect animals in Quebec. A few years after her death, the law was passed. I was so proud of her. She had made a difference!

As my lovely daughter always said, "You can change anything, you just have to believe."

Annabelle had very good grades in school. She was in a science program because she dreamed of becoming a veterinarian. Her favorite hobby was writing poems, and she was so good at it. She loved to write about her most intimate feelings. One day I told her, "You could be a reporter, a journalist, or even an author."

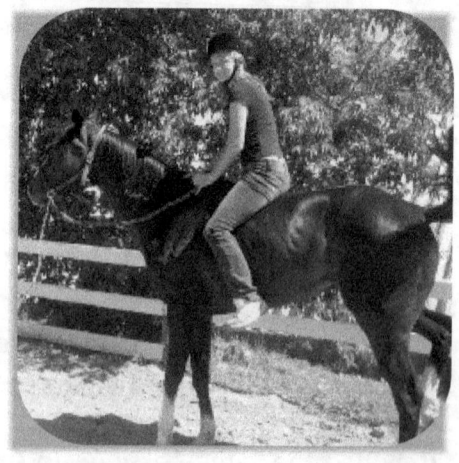

Annabelle was a girl with a lot of heart. She helped me take care of my mother. Mom lived next door, so when I prepared meals Annabelle would bring her one. She used to do a lot of little things for her.

Mom adored Annabelle and she was good for her. When we had family reunions, Annabelle always participated by helping prepare the meal and welcome the family. She enjoyed being with the family.

One day at a medical appointment when Annabelle was twelve years old the doctor talked to us about a new vaccine that would protect her from cancer. She would be cancer free. The vaccine was Gardasil. Until then, it was very important for her not to be sexually active.

My first reaction as a mother was to make a deal with her that there would be no boyfriend before she was 15-years-old, at least not before the vaccine. She agreed, even though at that time she didn't care about boys. But still, since Annabelle had given her word, I knew that she would wait. How lucky we thought we were to have this possibility to prevent cancer.

The summer of 2008, Annabelle was 14. My father and she rescued a horse from the slaughter house. The owner was unable to give him the care he needed to cure his foot that was in bad shape.

Since Dad had retired from the race horse business for 2 years, they both took on the responsibility of caring for Truck (that was its name). At the same time, it was a way for my father to be again closer to Annabelle. Truck could hardly walk. They spent the whole summer rubbing and walking the horse to give him a better life. Finally, after a few months of tender, loving care, just before starting school, he had recovered to the point where she could actually ride on his back. She was so proud. It was an emotional moment. My father and I cried just looking at her eyes.

When school was about to start someone else took Truck under their wings. Annabelle was getting news about him once in a while and knew that he was getting good care. Ironically Truck survived Annabelle. My Dad had him put to sleep 2 years after Annabelle death.

So her 3rd year of high school began. Annabelle was very happy in her new school and was especially thrilled to see all of her friends again.

The school nurse talked to us about Gardasil. It was going to be administrated during the year, but no date was determined. In Quebec, the medical law states teenagers at 14-years-old are free to make their own decisions regarding all medical matters without telling their parents.

On the night of October 24th 2008, she came out of her room completely disoriented, was speechless and had no coordination. I was in shock. I didn't understand what was happening to her. After 45 minutes trying to just have her say a word without mumbling, she slowly came back to herself. It was like if she had lost all her brain functions for a short time.

We rushed to the emergency room. She was on observation all night and the next morning she had a CT scan that came out normal.

I remember holding her hand that night and telling myself that if anything ever happened to her, I would die.

We went home and life got back to normal as if the incident had never happened.

That is, until the night of December 9th, when she went to take her bath at 7 pm with her book under her arm as usual. After 20 minutes I asked her if she was OK.

I have to say that Annabelle was old enough to take her bath alone, but I always asked instinctively if she was OK. My fear was that she might fall asleep while reading her book. I may add that it was forbidden to take her bath when she was alone in the house.

That night, my worst nightmare became a reality. There was no answer. I immediately panicked. I knew something was wrong. I asked again and still the silence. Finally, I unlocked the door and found her under water, eyes opened. I stopped breathing... I got on my knees and tried to take her out of the bath, but was unable to do so. I opened the front door and yelled so hard at Michel. He was shoveling snow in the driveway. We managed to take her out of the bath and lay her down on the floor. My first reflex was to try to wake her up. She had no response.

Michel called 911, I guess. My neighbour came to help. Then the paramedics took me away from

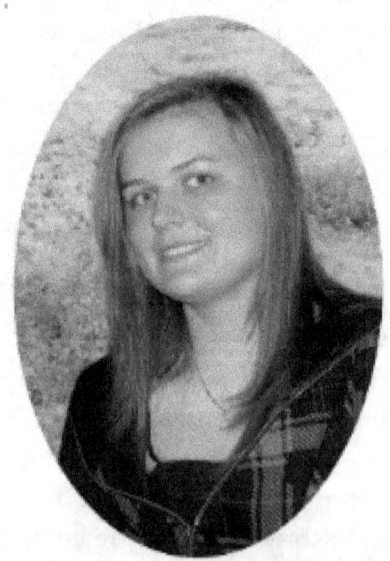

The last photo taken of Annabelle, 26 hours before she left this world.

her. Everything was going so fast, but at the same time I could feel my life crumbling down under my feet.

It was the worst nightmare of my life and I couldn't get out of it. She was brought to the hospital and they informed me that she came in with a cardio respiratory arrest. It took me a few minutes to realise that she had passed and that she wasn't coming back home with us.

At that precise moment a thick veil covered my eyes. Everything became blurry and any information was delayed before getting to my brain.

I remember telling my father: *"Look at her, because it's the last time you see her."* I just couldn't imagine seeing her in a coffin. She was going to be cremated.

There are moments when I think about them that I can still feel the intense pain. Once again, I experience how my heart felt when the doctor gave me her belongings in a pill bottle. There was her gold chain with the horse shoe, and a gold playboy rabbit in diamonds, a jewelry piercing from her belly button. That was all there was left of my healthy daughter after the night of December 9th 2008.

The night Annabelle passed it felt like a bomb had exploded in our family. The explosion was so violent it shattered fragments on every member of our family. Some bigger than others, some more painful than others, but all of them accompanied by memories we will never forget.

Nobody understood what had happened to Annabelle. We were in shock. My daughter was in perfect health except the incident in October when they didn't find anything abnormal. But this time, nothing would ever return to normal. I stopped drinking when Annabelle was 17-months-old. I stopped for her sake; when she passed away, naturally I considered drinking again. But my first thought was: *I stopped for her - there is no way I'm going to start because of losing her.*

To this day, it's still very emotional and demanding for me to think back and talk about the darkest minutes, hours, days, weeks, months and years following that night. Believe me, at the beginning, you feel every single agonizing moment. At times the pain is so intense you simply forget to breath.

I remember getting up in the morning and sitting down in the rocking chair, just crying from inside, tears falling down my cheeks continually and Michel making me cups of coffee one at the time and just listening to me. Waiting for me to get just a bit better.

I couldn't sleep, so I naturally started sleeping in Annabelle's room, to feel closer to her, I guess. The first month Michel stayed beside me till I fell asleep. I slept in Annabelle's room for almost 7 years.

I remember shaking my head in the morning saying to myself *it's impossible, she's going to come out of her room.* I had to make an effort every morning just to get out of bed and move to the rocking chair. I knew I had to at least try to eat breakfast and a bit at dinner to survive. It was so hard for me to try and stay alive. I could feel my heart aching and empty; I wanted to die.

I was so mad at Michel for still having his children. I was a mess. One morning I thought about my parents. I knew that I had to be stronger for them and at least try my best to survive this. They had lost their son, as my brother Alain died at age 21 of a car accident. I had to be strong. At that precise moment, I knew I had to get better. Every time I was around Mom or Dad I would make the biggest effort to look in control. It was very difficult because I wasn't honest with them, but I felt that I had to spare them. Then they became my first stone to rebuild my new life as an orphan mother.

December used to be the best month of the year for our family. We had my birthday on the 17th, that year Annabelle had her autopsy, and then Christmas came shortly after. I don't remember Christmas except that the Christmas tree was not there in the morning (Michel had put everything away during the night of the 25th). Instead of celebrating Annabelle's 15th birthday on the 26th of December, family, friends, teachers, neighbours celebrated her funeral. The church was full. I don't remember much.

Michel was always there by my side, I know, but it's funny because the only moments I remember him during this time is in the mornings. It must have been so difficult for him, not having his wife beside him all that time. Yet every morning he was there full of compassion waiting for me to get out of Annabelle's room, hoping I was a little bit better, ready to sit down and listen to me and holding me in his arms when I was out of control crying my heart out. I love that man so much.

Death works in so many ways. Part of the family got closer and part of it just left us alone with our grief. After 10 years now, I have to say that the ones that stayed or got closer are now what I call *my heart family.*

Two months after Annabelle passed away, there was an article in the newspaper about three girls being hospitalised after receiving shots of

Gardasil. At that precise moment I remembered she was supposed to get the vaccine during the year. I immediately called the school, asked them if Annabelle had received Gardasil and if so, I needed to know the dates of the shots.

The first one was on October 9th and the second one, on November 24th.

My head began spinning as I realised that both shots were given 15 days before each medical event. In my mind, it was clear: Gardasil had done this to Annabelle.

This realization marked the beginning of a difficult journey for all of us. When I was finding information and medical papers on the chronology of the events, sometimes I had the feeling I was bringing her back to life. It was almost like some piece of information I might find could save her.

One day, I said to myself *Ok stop, you can't save her. It's too late. She is not coming back.* Then I fell apart. I had so many documents and papers proving it was chronologically without a doubt the vaccine.

So I filed a lawsuit against Merck, and the doctors and nurses who were involved in Annabelle's last 2 months of life, from October 9th to December 9th 2008. Two months, that's what it took to take her life, her future and her dreams. Sadly in Quebec, you need a doctor to represent you in court who is willing to state the vaccine is responsible for at least 51% of the death. I tried for 7 years to find one. After 55 thousand dollars spent and exhausting our physical and emotional energy, I gave up.

During all these years and still today, I do my best to warn others about side effects possible after HPV vaccinations. New symptoms can appear up to several months after the shots have been administered. I make sure that young boys and girls know they can refuse to get the second shot if they have a problem after the first injection.

The anniversary dates of Annabelle's HPV vaccinations are a nightmare for our family. We have to force ourselves not to succumb to reliving the pain. No family needs to go through what we did.

Grief works in a funny way. In the beginning, we would always avoid talking about Annabelle at family reunions because we would all start crying. Everyone missed her so much. So, everyone handled their grief in their own way. Family reunions were very hard for me. The only thing I saw was my daughter's empty seat. So, I stopped going to birthdays, family dinners, and any events that would make me think about my loss.

Then, just when I needed it most, a special friend come back into my life. Caroline had lost a baby two years prior to my daughter's death. At that time she had one baby girl named Rose and was pregnant with Veronique. Our shared loss helped us become very close to each other. I started visiting her at her home twice a week, holding her baby, putting her to sleep in my arms, just looking at her and remembering Annabelle. I believe that we grieved together our lost ones. It must have been very hard for her to relive her own pain. But, Caroline's home was my safe place where I felt understood, a shelter where I could let go and cry and still feel loved. I said many times that these three special human beings saved my life and they will always be part of my existence.

In the beginning it was tough every day. It took a lot of time for my mind and body to understand what had happened.

I remember at the beginning of September 2009, Annabelle's school bus passed in front of the house. I went to the window and started waiting for her. It was the first day of school. I even said to myself *she must have stopped at her best friend house to talk about their first day* and then reality hit me like a ton of bricks. I crashed down on the floor. My legs couldn't support me. I screamed and realised that she wasn't coming back. I went to find Michel outside, looked at him and screamed so loud telling him *Annabelle will never come back.*

He held me in his arms for 10 minutes and we cried together, I believe, for the first time. One month later, I went to the emergency room for a panic attack. I could hardly breathe. They put me on medication and I started therapy.

Through the years I had three therapies and Michel had one, because he had been forgetting about his own needs. His life was only about getting me better. Sometimes I wonder how he managed to be there every day, always by my side. One day he told me *how can I ask you to comfort me? I just can't imagine your pain. It must be 100 times worse than mine.* Even so, I knew that he loved her as his own.

One day, at the beginning of my 3rd therapy, the therapist started our first appointment by telling me, "I have a pill that will take all your pain and sadness away, but it will also take away all souvenirs of Annabelle as if she never existed in your life. Do you want it?"

I started crying, without thinking, and naturally I answered, "My souvenirs are the only things that's left of her and I never want to forget her. She is part of me and will always be."

This moment started a new approach for me. I started thinking more about happy moments with Annabelle and wanted to talk about her more often. I quickly realised that talking about her was keeping her alive. It wasn't easy at the beginning for my family but it made sense for me.

For Mom and Dad it was particularly hard, I could feel their pain as they listened to me. My other heart sister, Marie-José, is very spiritual and helped me a lot in her own way, and always made me feel better. One day she told me a phrase of hope that I always think about, *"Every step you make, you get closer to Annabelle."*

I remember when the first anniversary of Annabelle's death was approaching. I was starting to fall apart again and my therapist told me, *"You know Linda, for you, every day is the 9th of December. So no need to anticipate."* He knew exactly how I felt every day.

So I decided to do something special. Something symbolic. I got a tattoo on my heart representing her. A horse shoe with two angel wings and her lucky number 2. Nobody knew my intention. Finally Michel, my best friend Ginette and my Dad had tattoos done also. On Mother's Day, Mom had 2 roses with wings tattooed on her heart. The five of us got tattooed for the first time in our lives. It was good for our grief process. It made us closer and we all felt closer to Annabelle.

Today, I'm sure of one thing: everyone in the family could write their own story about Annabelle's death and each one of them would be tragic. Michel and I lost our daughter. My parents lost their granddaughter. Michel's children lost their sister. One lost her Godmother. Some, their loved cousin. Others, their niece. Others, their best friend. Annabelle represented all this. Her passing has left an empty space in everybody's heart and life.

It's very difficult when you realise that you won't be excited for your daughter at her high school prom; you will never meet her first boyfriend; you will never get to marry her to the man of her life; and, you will never experience the joy of becoming a grandmother. But must important, you will not have her by your side as you grow old.

When I was pregnant with Annabelle, I remember thinking to myself: *I will never be alone anymore.*

Now, not only will she NOT be here, she left an emptiness in my heart that is always there. Life itself makes me remember the pain. When it happens it's just as intense as at the very beginning.

The last weekend of Annabelle's life, we had the chance to go shopping for her first young lady Christmas dress. It was a special event, something very important for her. I will always cherish these hours together. We had so much fun. She was trying on high heels for the first time and

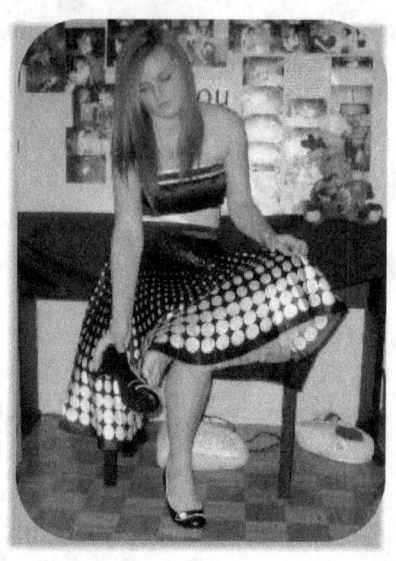

could barely walk in them. It makes me smile just writing it. She found a beautiful black and white dress. When she tried it on, I then realised my little daughter was now a young woman. I was so proud of her.

The day before she passed, she had her friend home to show her dress and they took pictures, so many pictures of her in that dress. She was so happy she could hardly wait for Christmas. Sadly she never had the chance to wear it. I couldn't give it away after. So it stayed in her closet, where it remains today.

On July 26, 2009, we did Annabelle's burial. It was the date of my brother Alain's birthday. Every year since Annabelle was born, we used to go to Alain's grave and bring him flowers. Every year, I would take a picture of her beside the stone. This is the last picture I took at the grave with Dad, Annabelle and I in 2008. The next year at the same date, I couldn't believe that Annabelle's name was under Alain's name on the stone. She used to sign Annabelle Mor, so I decided to have it engraved on the gravestone. That's what she would have wanted.

Through the years I have found ways to feel her close to me. I keep some of her belongings that were significant for her. When I travel I always take with me her last school backpack, and her stuffed horse Spirit in my luggage. The first thing I do when I get in my hotel room is to take a picture of Spirit on the bed. Spirit stays with me every night during my vacation. A second thing Annabelle had started was to collect keychains on her backpack. So, everywhere I travel I find one that I believe represents her. I think that when you are grieving you have to do whatever works for you.

Her lucky number 2, the 9th of her death and the 26th day of her birth are three numbers that are always around me. Every time they appear in different situations, I take it as a sign of her presence. I have to say that there is no time limit prescribed during which to handle your grief. For me, after seven years, I was feeling better and wanted more to live. I wanted to live for both of us: Annabelle and I. My daughter had so many dreams.

In January 2015, I started to really take care of myself. I began exercising five days a week. I lost 60 pounds in a healthy way. My partner and I were doing so well that we decided to get married after 20 years together. The date of the wedding was highly symbolic and chosen on purpose: we decided it would be on July 26th. For us, this decision symbolised a new beginning without forgetting the past. We felt like we were uniting forever our lives with each other and Annabelle. In my wildest dream, I would never have thought that Annabelle's Christmas dress would fit me. But after losing so much weight, I couldn't resist trying it on. It fit me perfectly! The precious souvenir of that happy day with my girl was brought back to my present life. So I got married in Annabelle's Christmas dress. I felt her with us all throughout that day. I have to say everything was about Annabelle that day. She was our honored guest at the ceremony and through the whole event. She guided us every step of the way throughout the day. It was celebrated in my yard, beside Annabelle's lilac with my heart family. Everybody was happy for us that we were able to look forward to a new future together. Even if I was 55 years old. I believe we took a burden off my parent's shoulders that day: their girl could finally be happy again.

For sure I would have loved having Annabelle with us. Years taught me that I have to remember my happy years as a mother. When I think of her, I always see her at 2-years-old, sometimes at 6 or 14-years-old. I try hard not to think of her as she might have been in the future that was robbed from us. It's too hard for my soul.

As I write these lines, it comes to my mind that she would be 25-years-old this December 26th 2018. She would probably have been accepted as a veterinarian or a journalist or even been known for her new bestseller book. She would also be probably having a baby soon. Some of her friends are already mothers. It makes me think that I would have been a very proud grandmother...the more I think about it, the more it hurts. As soon as the emotion kicks in, I have to stop thinking about this now inaccessible dream.

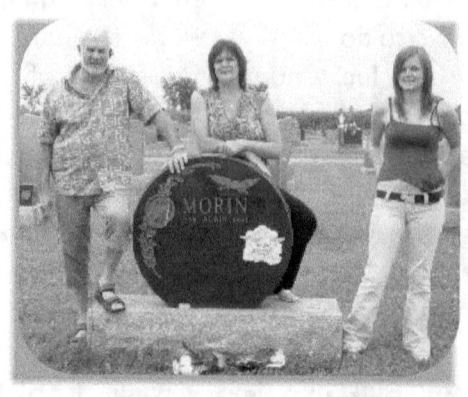

Mom passed away last year, and another grief came along. It was hard. But I remember the thought I had when it happened. I was happy for her. Her loneliness was finally over. She had grieved for her son, then for her granddaughter. I hoped and wished so much that Annabelle was there guiding her to heaven so she could finally be reunited with her son Alain. I know she was... She loved her Mamy so much.

Since Annabelle's death, Michel and I take an hour each morning to spend time with each other and talk about anything that's on our mind while we drink our 2 coffees together. One morning while having my morning coffee with Michel, I told him that if ever I had a cardiac arrest or anything that involved artificial resuscitation, especially if my parents were dead, to please let me go and refuse all extraordinary measures. I believe that Annabelle will be right there waiting for me, telling me, *"Come on Mom, follow me."* Being revived would make me so mad, for having been so close to her and not having the chance to take her in my arms again. I simply could not live with the loss one more time.

Now after 10 years, I have the privilege to be a godmother for the first time in my life, for a beautiful angel (our second gift of God in the family). My heart sister Sarah named her Arielle Annabelle in memory of her niece and to honor her. I was very moved by this gesture. My daughter won't be forgotten for a few more generations. They will be talking and remembering her; they will keep her alive. It's the best thing that has happened to me in a long time: her heart will still go on.

Ten years ago, by thinking that I was doing the right thing for my healthy daughter, believing that I was protecting her from cancer, her life was stolen. Exactly two months, from October 9th to December 9th: in so little time I lost my Annabelle. Her tragic story was short.

If only I knew...she would never have received these two shots of HPV vaccine. In spite of everything we have gone through, I am still pro-vaccine.

If I asked every member of my family how they feel about Annabelle's death ten years after this tragic event, they would all say with tears in their eyes that she will always be missed. That there is a before and an after December 9th. That she is still haunting our hearts and always will be.

Now, I understand my father and I are the ones who have suffered the most because of this tragedy. We are the most broken ones and we will never feel whole again. There is a big piece of our hearts missing. No matter how much time goes by, we still are very vulnerable.

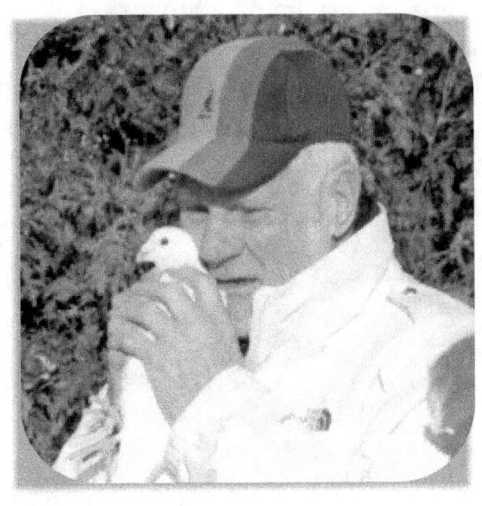

It is very important for me to honor and recognize my father for all the love he showed towards Annabelle through all the years and for the emotional support he offered me through all these years of pain. He always has been my rock and he still is.

It is still very difficult to express how my father and I feel about Annabelle's loss. This picture says it all. It was taken on Annabelle's 18th birthday at the cemetery, 4 years after she passed away. That day, every member of the family had a white dove in their hands to signify Annabelle's adult life and also, to free her soul symbolically. It was time to let Annabelle go free. But my father couldn't release the dove. He couldn't stop crying. It was unbearable.

This is exactly how we feel, each single day: we want to let go.....but we can't.

I have the chance that life brought me back Annabelle's cousin and best friend Maxime after eight years of absence. I believe his grief was so overwhelming that it took him all this time to be able to face the reality and accept his loss. A feeling, that I thought was buried long time ago, reappeared: I care about him like a mother. It's like Annabelle is living through him. I'm grateful for that relationship.

After Annabelle's death, three special girls also came into my life. I call them *Mes Poulettes*. They are a very big part my life as they help heal a part of my broken heart. They cure the motherhood in me that was wounded. Since Rose, Véronique and Arielle are very close to me, I can see my daughter through them. They make me smile again. I can remember Annabelle and live again pieces of what was taken from me.

Annabelle changed my life and is still doing so. I have been clean and sober for 23 years now. She is still my reason to stay sober and to live. The family is all doing better. We have to, if we want to survive this.

For me, every day is still a battle. My first thought in the morning is for or about Annabelle and she is the last thought before I close my eyes at night. I hope every night that I will dream of her. It's my only way left to see her. She has become my dream daughter.

Annabelle dreamed of reaching people through her writing. She wanted to change the world. By writing our story, I hope I'm granting her wish. Most importantly, by writing her story I am keeping her heart alive. I dearly hope she will always be remembered.

Mexico

HPV vaccines were introduced in Mexico in 2008, but only in 125 targeted communities comprising approximately 5% of the country's population. All of these communities were those of the 'lowest economical index' because it was assumed these communities had the highest incidence of cervical cancer. The quadrivalent HPV vaccine (Gardasil) was delivered to these communities via mobile health clinics. The targeted age group was girls, ages 12 to 16.[26] Coverage for the first dose was 98%. The completion rate for the 3-dose series was 81%.

In 2009, the program was extended to include 182 municipalities, also with the lowest human development index. The protocol for vaccine administration changed to a targeted age group of 9 to 12, with a dosing schedule of two doses administered 6 months apart, with the third dose given five years later.[27] According to Chapter 4 of the 'Comprehensive Cervical Cancer Control: A guide to essential practice,' published by the World Health Organization, this dosing schedule was not approved or recommended.[28] At the time, only 3 other countries were using alternative dosing schedules: Colombia, Switzerland and parts of Canada.[29] Nevertheless, coverage for the first dose was 85% with the second dose coverage coming in at 67%.

In 2011, Mexico's National Immunization Council approved a nationwide expansion of the HPV vaccination program to include a school-based HPV vaccination program aimed at all 9-year-old girls.

Two months before leaving office, in 2012, the current President of Mexico, Felipe Calderon announced HPV vaccinations would be mandatory for all 11 to 12-year-old girls. According to the president's announcement, this program targeted one million schoolgirls and an additional 200,000 girls who were not enrolled in schools. At the time, only one other country, Greece, had made HPV vaccines mandatory.[30]

---

[26] Progress Toward Implementation of Human Papillomavirus Vaccination---the Americas, 2006-2010; CDC; accessed March 2019

[27] ibid

[28] Comprehensive Cervical Cancer Control: A guide to essential practice; WHO; 11 February 2013; page 6; accessed March 2019

[29] Ibid ref 26

[30] Johnson, Tim; Mexico orders HPV vaccinations for all 5th grade girls, saying

When the current Minister of Health, Jose Angel Cordova, made the formal announcement in August 2011, the targeted age group had 'mysteriously' changed to age 9. His announcement included the statement, "Deaths from cervical cancer had fallen 47% during the last two decades."[31]

Evidently, he was referencing a 2008 article published in 'The Lancet' stating, "The decrease in cervical cancer mortality observed in Mexico is proportional to increasing Pap coverage and decreasing birthrate. Accreditation of cervical cytology laboratories is needed to improve diagnostic precision."[32]

Why did the Mexican government not decide to increase the public's access to Pap screening? One can only guess.

On December 21, 2014, Ximena M. died when she was only 14 years old, after two years of suffering that started with her second injection of Gardasil.[33]

May 2015, after only 500 doses of Gardasil were administered under Mexico's mandatory HPV vaccination program, the Mexican Social Security Institute (IMSS) had to cancel the HPV immunization program at some schools because parents were refusing to allow their 9-year-old girls to receive the injections.[34]

Did the parents in Mexico know something their government was not willing to disclose?

---

it will end threat of cervical cancer; McClatchy Newspapers; 3 Oct 2012; accessed March 2019

[31] Staff writer; Mexico to give HPV   vaccine to all girls from 2012; Agence France Press; 30 Aug 2011; accessed March 2019

[32] Decreasing Cervical Cancer Mortality in Mexico: Effect of Papanicolaou Coverage, Birthrate, and the Importance of Diagnostic Validity of Cytology; cEduardo Lazcano-Ponce, Lina Sofía Palacio-Mejia, Betania Allen-Leigh, Elsa Yunes-Diaz, Patricia Alonso, Raffaela Schiavon and Mauricio Hernandez-Avila; Cancer Epidemiol Biomarkers Prev October 1 2008 (17) (10) 2808-2817;**DOI:** 10.1158/1055-9965.EPI-07-2659; accessed March 2019

[33] Capilla, Alicia; AAVP: outraged by Mexican Girl's Death after HPV Vaccine; SaneVax Inc.; 10 Dec 2015; accessed March 2019

[34] Capilla, Alicia; HPV Vaccines: Updates from Central and South America; SaneVax Inc.; 13 June 2015

Please, let us wake up from the nightmare

By Mara Mexia, from Mexico

Six years ago today, in February 2013, I made a decision that I have regretted every day since. I remember it as if it had happened yesterday.

We went to the hospital to get the last dose of the HPV vaccine Gardasil for my daughter. Shortly before entering Preventive Medicine, while we were sitting there waiting, Yael asked me not to make her get the vaccine, telling me that the previous dose had hurt a lot. When I close my eyes, I can still see her face covered with tears as she asked me to please not have her get it again.

I remember turning to her and saying, "It's for your own good, it's just a small prick in exchange for not getting cancer."

Today those words are deeply engraved in my soul. I took her inside, almost pulling her along, as she was crying. At the time, I felt that I was being the most responsible mother in the world. I was fulfilling my duty as a parent: to take her to get her shots on time, without fail, just as I had always done. I never imagined all the suffering that awaited her.

That decision was the beginning of our nightmare. Two days later she fainted for the first time. The fourth day after, she began to feel the pains that would never leave her. New medical conditions, progressive paralysis, unbelievable pain, muscle weakness, and seemingly endless medical tests became our new 'normal'. Everything began to grow like an enormous ball of snow that destroyed everything in its path: her health, her dreams, our family's tranquility, our hope...

Today, six years later, each time I open my eyes in the morning my wish is still the same, to be able to go back in time, to find that this was just a nightmare. I want to wake up one morning and hear Yael tell me that she does not feel any more pain, she can walk without fear of falling, and that today she feels fine.

In spite of everything, though some days she is more tired than others, every day she decides to fight, one day at a time until she is finally able to reach a better day and there is some real improvement.

My warrior daughter, I regret in my soul having put you in this situation. Forgive me. I love you.

The Adolescence Gardasil Denied Me

By Yael Mexico

This is my story of adverse reactions to the human papilloma vaccine: the post-vaccine HPV syndrome, a new medical condition that may appear after vaccination against the human papillomavirus.

For the last six years I have been suffering the consequences of the adverse effects of the HPV vaccine. February 2013, after the third injection of Gardasil, my pilgrimage through hospitals began.

It still feels like yesterday, that feeling of uncertainty and fear and feeling totally lost. On a day like today, the HPV vaccine changed my life from one day to the next; it brought me pain, abandonment and many other feelings.

All of a sudden my friends vanished. My days just were not the same. I stopped living and only thought about surviving one more day. I still feel confusion and nostalgia to see the past. Everything in my life has been transformed so drastically.

Little by little, the days turned into weeks, weeks into months and months into years. Some days have been more difficult than others but all have been full of pain and suffering. Having lived through the last six years, I cannot say that it is possible to get used to the pain. What IS possible is to learn to live with it and accept it.

When you live without the certainty of knowing when it will stop, you get used to some symptoms. Then new ones appear and you have to get used to them. With each new symptom you try to concentrate on the hope that one day you will be able to live without pain and have a normal life.

My family and I still do not know what future we are facing. I just wish I could go back in time. I have lived a third of my life with so much pain that I cannot even remember how it feels to be free of symptoms, for me there are only bad days and worse days.

This is not the life I imagined as a 17-year-old. I refused to share my videos but I have the right to share my story. It is necessary for parents to have a clear idea of what their daughters might face if they are part of the small minority that is negatively affected: Fainting (neuro-cardiogenic syncope), hypotension, tachycardia, Raynaud's phenomenon, fasciculations, involuntary shaking of the legs, hand tremors, loss of strength, difficulty walking, indescribable pain in every part of the body, day and night, even while you sleep. Entire days in hospitals, this and much more is what the adverse reactions to Gardasil imply.

We reported my reactions to the Secretary of Health, Pharmacovigilance in my country and to the pharmacist both in Mexico and in the United States. We hoped that they had a protocol for these cases. They did not have one. The response of health authorities was that these things happen in a small percentage of those who receive the vaccine. The pharmacist replied that he would contact pharmacovigilance. The only thing I have obtained from them is a folio. No one has contemplated what to do or how to help those affected by HPV vaccines.

It is always inhumane to accept the suffering of a few for the good of the majority. It is even more inhumane to leave those who are suffering without hope of treatment, without hope of a normal future.

EUROPE

Austria

The vaccination program in Austria is rather unique. Once a vaccine is licensed, it becomes available for individual use via private pay through pharmacies. From there, the Ministry of Health (MOH) asks the Supreme Health Council (OCS) to study the feasibility and suitability of including that particular vaccine in the National Immunization Program (NIP). The resulting report goes back to the MOH for analysis by their own vaccination expert committee and ultimately a final decision by the Minister of Health. If approval is granted for inclusion in the National Immunization Program, the vaccine becomes taxpayer funded. No vaccines are mandatory. Direct advertising of pharmaceutical products is not allowed.

The HPV vaccine Gardasil was licensed for use in both girls and boys in October 2006. At the time, Austria had a pap screening program, but no national structure in place to send out invitations to participate or reminders for future appointments. Participation in the program was estimated at around 30%.

By September 2007, the Supreme Health Council (OCS) issued a recommendation in favor of adding Gardasil to the national immunization program for both boys and girls. Now it was up to the experts from OCS and the vaccination experts within the Ministry of Health to convince the Health Minister, Andrea Kdolsky, that adding HPV vaccinations to the national schedule was prudent, perhaps even imperative.

The problem was Health Minister Kdolsky was a medical doctor with many concerns regarding the potential addition of Gardasil to Austria's National Immunization Program. She was skeptical about the use of the vaccine and thought adding it to the NIP might interfere with the already struggling Pap screening program. Unlike many others, she wanted evidence that eliminating a virus associated with cancer would have an impact on diagnosis rates. She wanted evidence-based data and long-term studies regarding the safety and efficacy of Gardasil before she subjected her citizens to a mass vaccination program. Dr. Kdolsky wanted to know what effect injecting genetically engineered virus-like particles (VLP's) would have on people. In addition to safety concerns, there were also budgetary issues. Gardasil would be an expensive addition to Austria's health care budget.

These concerns were echoed by several segments of her constituency. The debate between those with concerns and those who believed HPV vaccines were one of the greatest developments of the century raged on throughout the country.

As an elected official, Minister Kdolsky believed she had a responsibility to examine as much reliable data as possible before making a final decision. Therefore, for the first time in Austrian history, she commissioned a Health Technology Assessment to be conducted by a newly founded research institute. The institute would analyze each intervention (Pap versus HPV vaccines) considering safety, efficacy, effectiveness, necessity, economic efficiency, social impact, and equity. Their report was to only focus on economic evaluations and be filed with the Ministry of Health by the end of 2007.[35]

- The conclusion of the report left Minister Kdolsky three options:
- Improve the current screening program
- Implement HPV vaccination, but negotiate a lower price
- Implement HPV vaccination at the currently offered price

The Minister of Health chose to make HPV vaccines available in pharmacies for private purchase, but not included in the publicly funded National Immunization Program. This decision virtually put an end to the HPV vaccine debate in Austria, at least at the federal health policy making level.

---

[35] Paul, Katharina T.; "Saving lives": Adapting and adopting Human Papilloma Virus (HPV) vaccination in Austria; Elsevier BV; 6 Feb 2016; PMID 26921384; accessed March 2019

Needless to say, HPV vaccine stakeholders were not happy with this decision. They spent the next few years working to re-frame the HPV vaccine message. Every newly published study was used as evidence that HPV vaccines would 'save lives' and 'fight cancer'. These were two points no one wanted to argue with. Who wouldn't want to fight cancer and save lives?

Eventually, HPV vaccines were successfully re-branded as a public need rather than just a vaccine to prevent women from contracting cervical cancer. Now, anyone who dared question their use appeared to be irrationally acting against their own best interests as well as the best interests of Austrian citizens.

In 2012, a new Minister of Health took office. Minister Alois Stöger was thought to be in favor of HPV vaccine use. During 2012, two new vaccines were added to Austria's National Immunization Program against pneumococcal and meningococcal infections. Statistical surveillance of HPV infections and cancers associated with them was instituted. Officials at the MOH formed new collaborative networks with pharmaceutical manufacturers declaring their shared goal of promoting vaccine uptake. A new coalition called the Austrian Association of Vaccine Manufacturers was formed with the aim of promoting 'evidence-based political discourse on vaccination'. Campaigns were organized at selected events to generate support for the use of HPV vaccines. The message appeared to be 'vaccination is a responsibility, not only for individual protection, but to protect all of society'.

Evidence came in from Swiss trials indicating two doses, instead of three, offered adequate protection. This would make it easier to get children fully vaccinated during a single school year. At the same time, the price of Gardasil dropped dramatically. A new and improved Gardasil 9 was released, promising to cover a higher percentage of high-risk HPV types. The stage was now properly set.

In August 2013, Minister of Health, Alois Stöger, announced, "We have expanded the free children's vaccination program step by step. I am certain that, with the inclusion of the vaccine against HPV, we will be offering an essential contribution to the health of our children. We will save lives."

Evidently, Gardasil had to be adapted in order to be good enough for Austria. As of 2016, it was estimated that 50% of the boys and 40% of the girls in Austria had failed to receive the first dose of Gardasil.[36]

Apparently, half of Austrian citizens were not convinced that Gardasil was one of the best inventions since sliced bread.

---

[36] Borena, Wegene; Luckner-Hornischer, Anita; Katzgraber, Franz; Holm-von Laer, Dorothee; Factors affecting HPV vaccine acceptance in west Austria: Do we need to revise the current immunization scheme?; Elsevier BV; Dec 2016; PMID 29074178; accessed March 2019

No Causal Association Established?

Information submitted by Jasmin's parents, Austria

Jasmin was a lively, active, sporty 19-year-old girl. She had been educated in a high school for sports with a concentration on ergotherapy for disabled people. She did volunteer social work for 10 months at a secondary school in Norway. Jasmin also did volunteer work as an assistant in an institution for disabled people in upper Austria. She was a student of International Development at the University of Vienna.

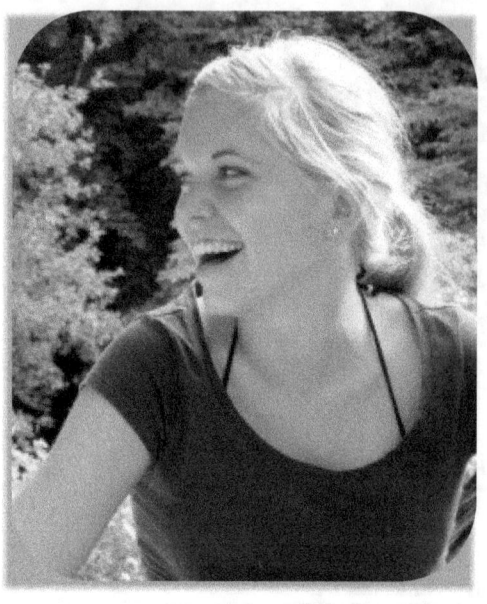

In short, Jasmin was fit, happy and fun-loving. She had never experienced any serious illnesses, had no history of lung disease and had never smoked. She had experienced no problems after any of her previous childhood vaccinations which were administered according to the recommended schedule.

Jasmin received her final injection of the HPV vaccine, Gardasil, on September 19, 2007. Twenty-three days later, on October 12, 2007, she was found dead. Apparently, she had died in her sleep.

Searching for answers, her parents meticulously reconstructed the final hours of her life. According to their investigation:

She was at a concert, a Spanish band. Before midnight, she was at a fast-food restaurant. She then rode with her flat-mate home, via taxi to Dobling. At approximately two o'clock in the morning, she drank some tea. The next morning, her girlfriend came by to check up on her, but according to her friend, "Jasmin must have died a few hours earlier in her sleep."

How could this happen to such a young, active, entirely healthy girl?

The autopsy confirmed she had no illness, no heart attack, and no problem with any of her internal organs. She had no injuries, no alcohol in her system, no drugs, no embolism, no viral or bacterial infections, nor was her death caused by an assault. The forensic physician concluded the cause of death was respiratory paralysis.

Expert Opinions:

Since Jasmin's death had occurred under unusual conditions, a formal investigation was required. This investigation would be conducted by forensic physician, Dr. Johann Missliwetz on behalf of the prosecutor's office.

At the time, Dr. Missliwetz was the Vice Chair of the Institute of Forensic Medicine at the University of Medicine in Vienna. He had worked for the Institute for nearly 40 years and had examined over 8,000 bodies post-mortem. His qualifications were impeccable as was his reputation.

Upon completion of his investigation, Dr. Missliwetz refused to rule out the possibility that Jasmin's death was related to her recent HPV vaccination. His final report filed for the prosecutor's office stated,

"Ultimately, it is the possibility of an allergic immunological event, or that the HPV vaccine was causally responsible for the onset of death, medically not ruled out."

Dr. Missliwetz also stated, due to the fact the judicial autopsy took place 6 days after her death proof could no longer be established. Dr. Missliwetz said a blood coagulation test could no longer be done because too much time had passed since Jasmin's death. Therefore, the immunological status of her blood could no longer be determined. From a medical point of view, it was too late to prove a causal link.

Dr. Missliwetz had conducted tests to determine if there was any evidence of drug or alcohol abuse. There was none. He also did not find evidence of a deficiency associated with any of her internal organs. He had discovered no evidence of foul play.

Therefore, he stood firm in his belief that an allergic immunologic occurrence could not be excluded, nor could it be ruled out that the HPV vaccination could have been causally associated with the respiratory paralysis which lead to Jasmin's death.

During a personal conversation, he mentioned that he suspected an inflammation of the nerves (ADEM) did not first attack Jasmin's non-essential nervous system, which would have presented with symptoms such as facial palsy, problems with her extremities, nausea, or a host of other potential issues. Instead, the inflammation immediately attacked a vital organ, in this case her lungs, resulting in respiratory paralysis.

As a forensic expert, Dr. Missliwetz was obliged by law to inform the authorities about the possibility that this death might have happened as a consequence of pharmaceutical treatment, namely the Gardasil vaccination.

From the day he made his report, he started to receive calls from colleagues urging him to change his opinion. They informed him 'this vaccine could save lives, but uptake would be negatively impacted if people believed there was a connection between Gardasil and Jasmin's death'. It did not seem to matter that broncho-spasms were mentioned in the vaccine information leaflet as a possible side-effect after Gardasil injections.

Dr. Missliwetz refused to alter his opinion.

In stark contrast to Dr. Missliwetz's report, other Viennese vaccine experts including gynecologist Elmar Joura, and Ingomar Mutz, Chair of the Vaccine Committee of the Supreme Council of Health, were quick to declare 'with almost certain probability' that the HPV vaccination had no causal connection with Jasmin's death. They claimed a vaccine reaction could not occur three weeks after vaccination.

All of this happened at the same time the European Medicines Agency (EMA) was investigating another death which had been reported in Germany shortly after a Gardasil injection.[37] The EMA's conclusion on both cases was:

The two European (death) cases were reported as part of the ongoing monitoring of drug safety. One occurred in Austria, the second in Germany, in both cases the cause of death could not be identified and no causal relationship could be established between the death of the young women and the use of 'Gardasil'.

An important point which was not stated in this EMA statement is the fact that there is a huge difference between no causal relationship being established and no causal relationship existing.

Nevertheless, because some of the Austrian experts doubted a connection between Gardasil and these two deaths, the EMA issued a statement claiming the benefit of HPV vaccinations continued to outweigh the risks.

---

[37] Prosecution closed proceedings, 'DerStandard', 1 Feb 2008

All of the experts involved in this case knew, or should have known, there are three essential parameters which confirm a potential causal relationship between death and a vaccine. These parameters are:

- A temporal association between the injection and death
- No other identified cause of death
- A biological plausible mechanism of action

The inflammatory autoimmune reaction described by Dr. Missliwetz which resulted in Jasmin's respiratory paralysis provides a biological plausible mechanism of action. The autopsy confirmed there was no other viable explanation for her death. Certainly, twenty-three days should be an acceptable 'temporal' association.

Dr. Klaus Hartmann is a German immunization expert who has been with the Paul Ehrlich Institute for the Scientific Assessment of Unwanted Effects of Vaccines for many years. In an article published in 'DerStandard' on the 19th of February 2008, he commented on the controversy surrounding Jasmin's untimely demise.[38] He stated her cause of death was presumed to be related to acute disseminated encephalomyelitis (ADEM).

According to Dr. Hartmann, this is one of the most common diagnoses in the vaccine damage cases he reviews in his own practice. He has found it to be one of the biggest problems associated with inactivated vaccines.

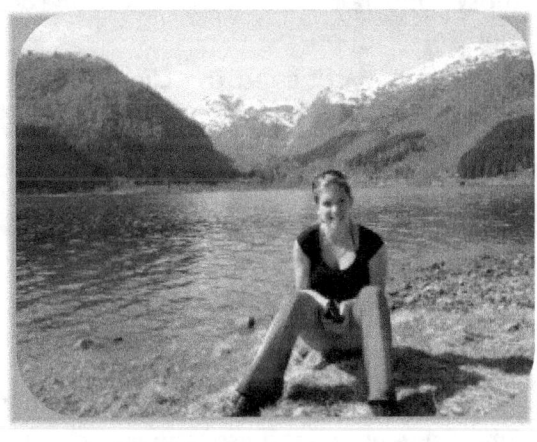

As an illustration, he pointed out another recent case of life-threatening inflammation of the nervous system (ADEM) which had been diagnosed in a 16-year-old girl three weeks after the HPV vaccine was administered. Luckily, her doctors recognized the condition because of

---

[38] Staff writer; HPV vaccine as a cause of death; DERSTANDARD; 19 Feb 2008; accessed March 2019

her blurred vision. They were able to save her via high-dose cortisone therapy.

Dr. Hartmann characterized ADEM as 'treacherous, fleeting, inflammatory events which often begin insidiously five to forty-two days after an infection or vaccination.

When speaking about Jasmin's case, he said,

> "She complained of headaches and severe intestinal problems. These are typical signs of ADEM. These symptoms indicate a fleeting inflammatory event, and if that happens in the respiratory center, respiratory arrest may result."

Dr. Hartmann said that statements like those of Vienna gynecologist Elmar Joura and Ingomar Mutz, chairman of the vaccination committee in the Supreme Medical Council claiming no causal association existed were 'complete scientific nonsense.'

Dr. Hartmann pointed out the fact that many vaccination experts have close financial relationships to HPV vaccine manufacturing companies.

He was also concerned about the HPV vaccine clinical trial protocols. Trials conducted prior to marketing authorization showed no conspicuous differences in the number of side effects experienced by those who received the HPV vaccine versus those who received the 'control' solutions.

Hartmann criticized the clinical trials of both Gardasil and Cervarix stating,

> "However, here, no neutral water solution was used as a placebo, but a mixture of the ingredients of the vaccine, including the proven problematic aluminum salts. As a result, any side effects were deliberately obscured."

According to Jasmin's father, Dr. Missliwetz was the only person who actively searched for the cause of Jasmin's death. All other entities up to the Ministry of Health only seemed interested in covering it all up.

After filing his formal report and refusing to alter his statement regarding the inability to rule out a causal association between Jasmin's death and Gardasil, one of Dr. Missliwitz's former colleagues was promoted to a position senior to Vice Chair Missliwitz.

Jasmine's father believes Dr. Missliwitz was subsequently harrassed, bullied and demeaned until he felt obliged to retire prematurely. Coincidence?

Denmark

In September 2006, the European Union licensed both Gardasil and Cervarix for use in males and females ages 9 through 26. Approximately one month later, Denmark licensed Gardasil use for females between the ages of 9 and 26. This made Gardasil available but only via private pay. During the next few years uptake rates varied substantially from one region to the next, ranging from a high of 33.1% to as little as 1.4% depending on location.

It was not until October 2008 that HPV vaccines were added to the Danish National Immunization Schedule making Gardasil free for all eligible females.[39] The first taxpayer funded HPV immunization program began in January 2009. Gardasil was offered to all girls who were at least 13-years-old. Several catch up programs were also conducted for girls ages 12 to 18. Uptake during the first year was 90% of those eligible, with 80% completing the 3-dose series. The uptake rates held fairly steady for the first few years.

In 2013, the situation changed. Suddenly there was a measurable drop in HPV vaccination rates. Newspapers, magazines and social media outlets began to report unusual new medical conditions manifesting after Gardasil injections.

In March 2015, a television documentary aired highlighting some of the Danish families who had experienced these new medical conditions. Over the next five years, Gardasil uptake declined substantially.

The wealthiest region of Denmark reported HPV vaccine uptake rates over the next five years as: 81% in 2012; 71% in 2013; 51% in 2014; 26% in 2015; and 13% in 2016.

---

[39] Charlotte Lynderup Lübker, Elsebeth Lynge; Stronger responders—uptake and decline of HPV-vaccination in Denmark, *European Journal of Public Health*; 8 Nov 2018; accessed March 2019

The lowest income region of Denmark was not much different. The reported uptake over the same period of time in this region were: 80% in 2012; 70% in 2013; 55% in 2014; 33% in 2015; and 16% in 2016.

By 2016, only 15% of Denmark's eligible female population was receiving the recommended number of Gardasil injections. This was despite the fact that Denmark had adopted a two-dose schedule in August 2009, making it much easier for girls and young women to complete the series at a substantially lower cost to the tax payers.[40]

The World Health Organization established a peer group in 2016 to help Denmark learn how to rebuild confidence in the HPV vaccination program based on the experiences of other European Union countries such as Ireland, the Netherlands and Austria.[41]

In 2017, the Danish Health Authority joined forces with the Danish Cancer Society and the Danish Medical Association to launch the 'Stop HPV, Stop Cervical Cancer' campaign. 'Public service announcements' became prominent in newspapers, magazines, social media outlets, and television.

According to an announcement made by the WHO in February 2018, less than nine months after Denmark's campaign was initiated, 31,000 eligible Danish females had received at least one HPV vaccination versus only 15,000 the previous year.

Nevertheless, the HPV vaccine controversy continues.

---

[40] Camilla Hiul Suppli, Niels Dalum Hansen, Mette Rasmussen, Palle Valentiner-Branth, Tyra Grove Krause, Kåre Mølbak; Decline in HPV-vaccination uptake in Denmark – the association between HPV-related media coverage and HPV-vaccination; BMC Public Health, 2018, Volume 18, Number 1, Page 1; 10 Dec 2018; accessed March 2019

[41] WHO: Denmark rebuilds confidence in HPV vaccination; Feb 2018; accessed March 2019

Betrayed and Abandoned

By Hans Friis Lauszus, Kolding, Denmark

I am the father of five children. Our family lives in a large waterfront home on Kolding Fjord in Denmark. We enjoyed a normal life in beautiful surroundings until we experienced what global health authorities say is a 'one in a million' chance – vaccine injury. My youngest child, a son, was injured by Pandemrix. His sister was injured by Gardasil. How could something so rare hit the same family twice?

Astrid is my fourth child. She was a happy girl with a lot of friends and had a non-eventful upbringing. In short, she was a normal child who enjoyed life.

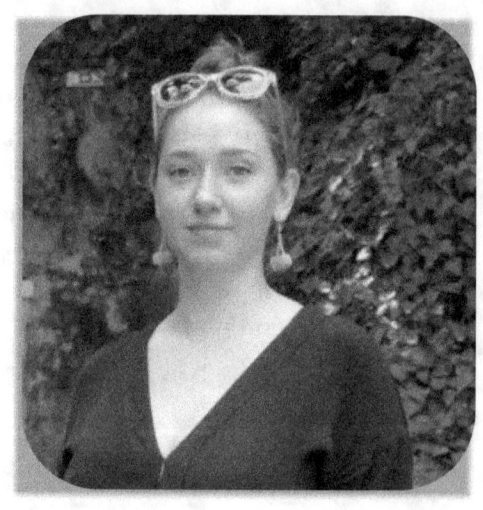

When Astrid turned 12-years-old in 2009, she got her Gardasil jab. Her mother had experienced serious cervical infections which required surgery. Consequently, we as parents did not question the vaccine at all. We were simply doing what was necessary to protect our daughter.

Astrid's first reactions to the Gardasil vaccine were rashes, skin problems, bruises, headaches and a great desire to sleep all day long. We thought nothing of all this. Our family doctor was not concerned either. The new symptoms were all classified as normal teenage behavior and puberty issues.

However, her symptoms increased in force. Ultimately Astrid was unable to walk and was forced to stay in bed due to extreme headache, hypersensitive to light and sounds. She was now losing skin from her hands, fingers and feet. We were in shock.

We were certain that we would be supported by the national health service of Denmark because the symptoms were clearly so severe that puberty could not explain them.

In spite of the fact that by this time there was a lot of media coverage in Denmark and other countries identifying problems with the Gardasil vaccine, our family doctor continued to label her symptoms as anything other than a vaccine injury.

Having seen her brother go through hell with Pandemrix, we as Astrid's parents reached out to other Danish parents who were convinced that their girls were injured by Gardasil. We were desperate to find Astrid the help she needed.

We were guided to a courageous family doctor by the name of Stig Gerdes, who at that time was the only one who had the guts to raise the alarm and speak up against Gardasil.

Astrid did a Melisa test, which showed a high response to Gardasil.

We knew from that moment on, this would be a lifelong battle against the public health, the patients' compensation fund and the media, which apparently is so sponsored by medical manufacturing companies, that they have sold their soul.

Astrid joined the association HPV injured daughters in Denmark and was guided to change her diet. She also learned to accept the fact that this injury would take a long time to get better.

After a seven-and-a-half year battle, Astrid received a diagnosis of ME and Pots from Professor Jesper Mehlsen at the Frederiksberg Synkopecenter. Finally, we had something concrete to deal with instead of simply a list of mysterious new medical problems.

Astrid had to leave high school 6 months before graduation, as she had too many absences from school and was unable to catch up due to fatigue. She was slowly recovering and we planned a gradual school restart in August 2017. But, Astrid's journey to regain her health took much longer than we anticipated.

Her body and general health were on a roller coaster ride for the rest of 2017 and first half of 2018. It was as if her body was desperately trying to recover, but could not get to a point where her power and mind could get the upper hand.

Astrid felt disappointed and isolated much of the time. She was unable to attend any meetings or social activities due to her condition. She had only 2 friends left. The rest had abandoned her due to them leaving for university or having boyfriends to go out with.

It is very hard to watch your daughter being isolated in this way, but we could not do anything to help.

The major shift came in May 2018, when she got high-dose vitamin C IV injections. That was a game changer!! Her body responded extremely well. The energy she got from vitamin C was enormous. Because Astrid had followed all recommendations in respect to detoxing, vitamins and mineral supplements, we believe her body was 'ready' for that energy boost.

Astrid got 12 IV vitamin C injections and her body and mind started to function again. She was able to respond rationally. She was able to think. She was able to read and UNDERSTAND what she was reading. She was able to go for longer walks and be social with her remaining 2 friends.

Wow! This was a cause for celebration!

It is very difficult to describe the ordeal we as parents have been through. Watching your child make the journey from being a happy 12-year-old girl to a 15-year-old zombie is no fun. I can only imagine how difficult it must have been for Astrid to have more than a third of her life ripped away.

On the bright side, Astrid has once again started on her high school education (restarted from 0). She can follow school and attend family activities. However, she has to follow a strict diet, take her vitamins and mineral supplements and rest when she feels she needs to, otherwise she will get too exhausted and her body will complain.

As parents and taxpayers, one of the biggest 'eye openers' for us was the total absence of support from our health system. We had already experienced life with a vaccine-injured child. We knew what was happening to Astrid shortly after her symptoms began to increase in intensity and diversity. We quickly realized what was to blame.

Did our health system support us? No!

Did our health system work to find out what was wrong with our daughter? No!

Did our health system try to find treatments for our daughter? No!

According to the medical system, our daughters were either having mental problems or were victims of coincidence. They had no medical issues, certainly none connected to Gardasil injections.

Not only that, our family and many others like us were treated as if we were idiots and subversives. How dare we question their authority? How dare we question the safety of this vaccine?

We were left feeling betrayed and abandoned; like the health system has sold its soul to the pharmaceutical industry and we, the people are doomed.

We have witnessed all of the suffering and pain our daughter has gone through. We have met many other young girls in similar circumstances. We cannot understand why this HPV madness is allowed to continue.

We demand a time-out until HPV vaccines are thoroughly tested.

France

There are two HPV vaccines available for use in France. Gardasil was approved in 2007 followed by the approval of Cervarix the following year. Both are available privately with 65% of the purchase price reimbursed by the National Health Insurance Program. The targeted group is females age 14, with catch-up programs available for females age 15 to 23. HPV vaccines are not mandatory in France, simply recommended.

Despite a rather good uptake in the targeted group during the first year (2007-50.8%), the rate of reimbursement for at least one dose in 2008 was only 41.7%. 2009 was even more dismal. The HPV vaccine was only injected in 20.5% of the targeted population that year. Remember, this was only 1 dose of a three-dose series. Nevertheless, by 2008 reimbursements for Gardasil were the fifth largest expenditure in the French National Health Insurance Program.[42] Health officials were beginning to question whether or not HPV vaccines were a wise investment considering the fact that cervical cancer screening was still needed despite vaccination status.

That was only the beginning of the controversy over HPV vaccines in France. Based on findings of making multiple false claims while advertising Gardasil in France, the Director General of the French Agency for the Safety of Health Products (AGSSAPS) banned advertising of Gardasil in 'any form of information including canvassing, prospecting or indirect inducement to promote the prescription, sale or consumption' of the vaccine. This decision was handed down on the 31st of August 2010.[43]

---

[42] Fagot JP, Boutrelle A, Ricordeau P, Weill A, Allemand H.; HPV vaccination in France: uptake, costs and issues for the National Health Insurance; Elsevier; J. Vaccine; 27 April 2011; PMID 21382486; accessed March 2019

[43] Legifrance database; Decision of 31 August 2010 prohibiting an advertisement for a medicinal product mentioned in Article L. 5122-1; SASM 1020221S; accessed March 2019

In 2012, a committee composed of members of the French Parliament issued the results of their analysis aimed at answering whether Gardasil was a good way to fight cancer. Their final report must have been quite a disappointment to HPV vaccine stakeholders. Instead of confirming the recommendations of their national health authorities, the committee recommended stalling the distribution of Gardasil pending the completion of a more comprehensive risk-benefit analysis.[44]

Parliament appointed a group of immunologists and other researchers to find out more about Gardasil's long-term efficacy and what the most prudent target population would be in addition to basic questions regarding the safety of the vaccine. The group was also charged with determining whether those using HPV vaccines would be more likely to forgo normal gynecological screening because they believed they were protected from all risk of cervical cancer.[45]

Meanwhile, things were not going so well for HPV vaccines in the civilian sector. Young girls were beginning to experience new and sometimes debilitating medical conditions after HPV vaccine administration. Girls were experiencing tingling in their limbs, dizziness, chronic exhaustion, muscle spasms, seizures, vision/hearing/speech problems and autoimmune disorders including lupus, Guillain-Barre, multiple sclerosis. Many found themselves confined to wheelchairs. Claims for compensation were filed.

By the end of 2013, 49 families with daughters suffering from various autoimmune conditions after Gardasil injections had filed criminal complaints against Sanofi Pasteur, the marketing authorization holder for Gardasil in France.[46] As of June 2014, the number of families participating in litigation had risen to 100.[47]

The public and many government officials were beginning to wonder how ethical it was to put healthy young French women at risk of experiencing debilitating new medical conditions, or even death, in an

---

[44] Cuneo, Louise; Cervical Cancer-MPs put vaccine under observation; LePoint Health; 19 March 2012; accessed March 2019

[45] Niland, Kurt; Gardasil Distribution Stalled In France Pending Government-Ordered Study; Righting Injustice; 21 March 2012; accessed March 2019

[46] **Xaillé**, Anne; Gardasil: the impatience of families in the face of judicial silence; Le Journal des Femmes; updated 02/03/2015; accessed March 2019

[47] Kimball-Brooke, Helen; Spotlight on Gardasil in France; SaneVax.org/30 June 2014; accessed March 2019

effort to try and prevent a disease that may, or may not, manifest decades down the road. The question was particularly troubling in view of the fact that cervical cancer could be avoided in most cases by an already proven safe and effective method. Were HPV vaccines truly worth the financial burden they placed on the French healthcare budget?

Was it possible that HPV vaccines were causing more harm than good?

By 2018, the HPV vaccine completion rate for 16-year-old girls in France dropped to only 19%.[48]

Do the following stories provide an explanation?

---

[48] Lefèvre H, Moro MR, Lachal J; The New HPV Vaccination Policy in France; letter to the editor; NEJM; PMID 29562152; 22 March 2018; accessed March 2019

Marie-Océane Bourguignon

By Jean-Jacques and Yveline Bourguignon

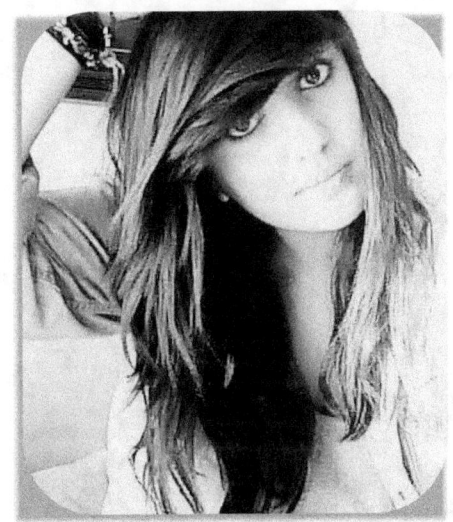

As Marie–Océane's parents, we publish our daughter's story hoping to help people realize there are potential risks involved with HPV vaccinations. We do not want anyone else to go through what we experienced without being aware of the possibility in advance.

Océane was a girl full of joy, health, and laughter before her 15th birthday. We affectionately called her our 'little pearl'. She never had to visit the doctor for an illness. That is until her life was turned upside-down because of trust. This is her story.

Océane was 15-years-old when she went to her family doctor to get a medical certificate for dancing with a friend. The doctor suggested Gardasil for cervical cancer prevention. We trusted our family doctor and consented to the vaccination. We did not realize this decision would set off a chain of events that would make Dante's Inferno look like a picnic.

In 2010, Marie-Océane Bourguignon, received two injections of Gardasil; the first on October 11th and the second on December 13th. Two weeks after the first injection, she experienced sensory and motor problems in her upper limbs before spontaneously and gradually regressing over a two-week period. We thought the tingling in her arms and loss of balance were simply a normal part of adolescence.

Two months later, after the second injection she vomited and suffered from severe dizziness. Three months after the second injection, on the 13th of March 2011, Marie–Océane was hospitalized for deterioration in her general health, cerebral-vestibular disturbances and sensory-motor impairment (ataxia-an inability to coordinate voluntary muscular movements), and vertigo.

On March 15, 2011, an MRI of her brain revealed lesions in the white matter. The year 2011 was a descent into hell for all of us. We spent our time traveling from home to hospital and back. Océane's attacks were devastating. She would appear to be in good health in the evening before bed and be vomiting as soon as she woke up the next morning. We didn't know from one day to the next what new symptom we would have to help Océane deal with.

We were very afraid of losing her because her last stroke left her in a wheelchair without vision or hearing due to the acute encephalomyelitis.

For two years, Océane could not attend school. Wheelchairs, facial paralysis, dizziness and great fatigue kept her home. Fortunately, she had friends to support her during the time she was suffering from so many new medical conditions.

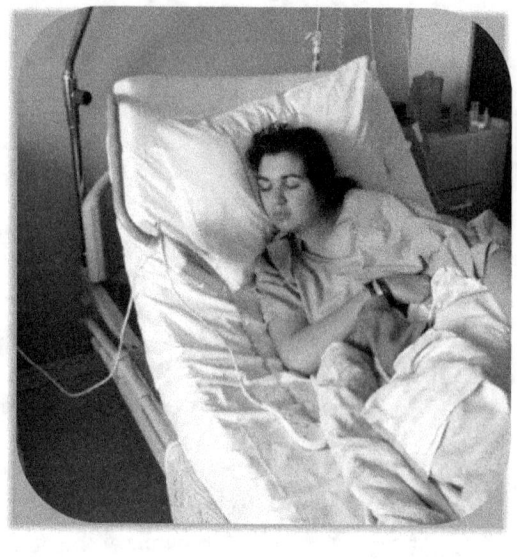

Her mother had to quit her job to be with Océane during her time of need. Yveline refused to leave our daughter alone when she was in such a physical and moral state. We lived in constant fear of losing our 'precious pearl'.

The doctors initially thought Marie was suffering from either multiple sclerosis or acute disseminated encephalomyelitis (ADEM). After many subsequent hospitalizations, it was thought she had developed multiple sclerosis, a chronic, typically progressive disease involving damage to the sheaths of nerve cells in the brain and spinal cord with symptoms including numbness, impairment of speech and muscular coordination, blurred vision, and severe fatigue. Marie-Océane will live with this condition for the rest of her life. There is no known cure.

Despite the fact her doctors hesitated to make a firm diagnosis for two years, they finally concluded she had encephalomyelitis (ADEM) which was a result of the HPV vaccinations. The temporal association between Océane's symptoms and Gardasil were quickly recognized by her doctors, who immediately filed a statement to pharmacovigilance regarding their assessment of the reasons for Marie's symptoms. That helped us avoid the medical wandering so many other French parents have been forced to endure when their daughters exhibited new medical conditions after Gardasil.

During the two years doctors were trying to decide on a final diagnosis for Marie, we requested an expert opinion from the Regional Commission for Medical Accidents in Aquitaine. They concluded that the pathology was consistent with a vaccine injury but that because her father (age 50) had type 2 diabetes, there was possibly an underlying genetic susceptibility.

Consequently, we filed for compensation on her behalf with CRCI, Regional Medical Injury Arbitration and Compensation Tribunal in Bordeaux on January 28, 2012.

In Bordeaux, on September 18, 2013, Judge Patrick Mairé handed down a decision stating Gardasil was 50% responsible for the permanent injury Marie's experienced after the two injections of the HPV vaccine she received. The other 50% was attributed to a genetic pre-disposition for autoimmune disorders.

Sanofi, which sells Gardasil on behalf of Merck in Europe had to make a compensation proposal. They did not accept accountability for the injury despite the first judgment and the reports of two medical experts. They remained in denial and alluded to the arrogance of our family for daring to claim our daughter's condition was a vaccine injury. Sanofi's settlement agreement even attempted to pass us off as anti-vaccine.

Even so, we were successful. We could have simply accepted the compensation award and gone on to try and rebuild our lives.

But we knew we were not the only ones to have had their lives turned upside down after Gardasil. We also knew the decision by CRCI would not be widely publicized, so others would not be warned about the potential risks involved with the use of HPV vaccines. We decided accepting the compensation would benefit no one other than our own family.

Consequently, we decided to turn down the award and take our case to a traditional criminal court where the outcome of any adjudication could be made public. We decided a just decision for our family was simply not good enough. We were determined to obtain justice for all victims of adverse events after Gardasil.

We knew there were more than 700 families in France who also had daughters suffering from serious new medical conditions after the administration of Gardasil (source: Agence Nationale Sécurité Médicament in France), but believed the health authorities hid it and minimized it with the complicity of the laboratories.

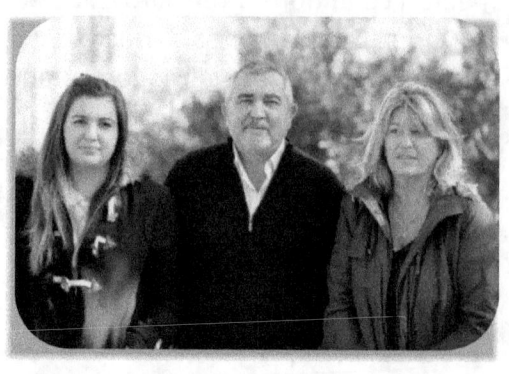

Faced with this injustice, we decided the only way we would have an opportunity to warn others was to take our case to the traditional court system for litigation. That would provide an opportunity to make the public aware of the fact that HPV vaccines can be quite dangerous for some individuals.

In November 2013, our attorney, Mr. Coubris, filed a criminal complaint against Sanofi Pasteur and the French Medicines Agency on behalf of our family and 50 other families like us.

In November 2015, we discovered this complaint had been buried by the Paris public prosecutor's office who stated there was no direct link between Gardasil and the pathologies of the nervous system experienced by the girls represented in Mr. Coubris' complaint. This was done without consulting any of the 50 families who had joined us in our criminal complaint.

None of us could believe the accountability of the vaccine had been established and yet the case was closed without our knowledge or an opportunity to be heard.

Attorney Coubris immediately filed an appeal and the families involved decided to also file a civil proceeding with the Dean of Investigating Judges in Paris.

Marie's life after injury

Today, Marie–Océane is still fighting to rebuild her life. At 20, she could not pursue her chosen career in architecture. At 22-years-old, she passed a pastry chef's CAP and wants to create her own business selling artisan pastries and local products. We hope she has a future in front of her, but realize it's not going to be easy.

She is still young, despite losing her teenage years. She will always be chronically ill and unable to work for a boss. In order to have a future, Marie will have to be her own boss so she can work at her own pace. Her parents will be behind her to help.

Our family continues to fight not only for our own daughter, but for all the other French families who are still suffering. We fight for the parents who have lost their children. We fight to help French families obtain justice for the sacrifices they have had to make simply because they trusted their doctors' advice.

We want the truth about this vaccine to be made public. We will accept nothing less than completely honest and open scientific debates. To accomplish this we enlisted the assistance of several independent associations to help facilitate symposiums on the subject within the medical/scientific community regardless of what the courts decide. We will not surrender.

Our daughter did not survive Gardasil

By Daniel K. from France

Our daughter Adriana died on October 20, 2010. She was only 17 years and 5 months old. This is her story:

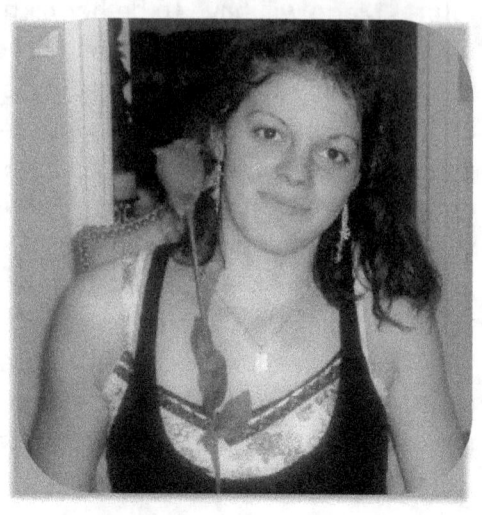

We will begin at the end, which is to say after her death because until then we did not know how our daughter had been struck down at such a young age. The multitude of examinations and tests she had undergone in the various hospitals where she had been admitted had not detected anything significant. Within the last three months of her life, from August until October 2010, Adriana had multiple diagnoses put forth including psychotic compensation, depression, catatonia, neuroleptic malignant syndrome, autoimmune disease, epilepsy, etc.... With no concrete test results to confirm these suspicions, we as parents were left in an overwhelming state of anxiety and distress. We needed answers.

Only one neurologist from the University Hospital of Toulouse who had followed Adriana's case to the end, had diagnosed Adriana without absolute certainty as having autoimmune encephalitis.

For these reasons, the hospital asked for our authorization for a post-mortem examination to be carried out in order to determine the cause of this 'inexplicable' death. Evidently, we were not the only ones looking for answers. Needless to say, we gave our consent.

It took nearly a year for us to get the results of the autopsy. In September 2011, we were informed that Adriana had died as a result of autoimmune meningo-encephalitis. This confirmed the diagnosis of her neurologist from the University Hospital of Toulouse, but provided no clue as to what caused the inflammation.

Annihilated by the pain and misunderstanding, we had to accept this verdict without being able to obtain further explanations.

In October 2011, quite by accident we discovered an article in the press about adverse effects of the Gardasil vaccine. It was a shock for us because some of the side-effects described were similar to those experienced by Adriana. After consulting the internet we were surprised by the large number of testimonials from others who had been devastated after using this vaccine.

We began to recall what it was like in 2008. At the time, there was a huge media blitz touting the benefits of Gardasil. We saw newspaper articles, posters in medical offices and clinics, signs in hospitals, all of them saying how wonderful this new vaccine was. It seemed everywhere you looked there was some sort of news article or public service announcement explaining how dangerous an HPV infection could be and how any responsible parent would want to protect their child from the ravages of cervical cancer.

In order to protect our daughter, and under the influence of the advertisements which were reinforced by her attending physician, we agreed to the vaccination. Unfortunately, we did not know at the time that this vaccination was already controversial.

After the first injection in October 2008, Adriana felt the first undesirable effects: headaches, stomach aches...nothing particularly alarming for a teenager.

These new symptoms became progressively much more prominent after the second injection on December 19, 2008. In addition, she began to have anxiety attacks, hot flushes, tingling in her legs, muscle pain, difficulty walking, hair loss, and other symptoms culminating in a significant syncope episode on April 18, 2009.

Adriana received her third injection of Gardasil on April 24, 2009. Once again, all of her previous symptoms continued intermittently while new ones appeared. Now, in addition to everything else, she was suffering from debilitating fatigue, fainting, severe mood swings, and loss of appetite.

None of these events seemed to worry her doctor. He advised us to consult a psychiatrist. It seemed he believed Adriana's problems were primarily psychological and that Adriana's fainting was a result of small vagal discomfort. The GP had ordered an electroencephalogram, but it had not detected anything in particular. In view of this, we continued to trust our GP. Therefore, we agreed to allow Adriana to consult with a psychiatrist. Unfortunately, this consultation had only detrimental effects.

On June 16, 2010, Adriana had a tonsillectomy and adenoidectomy. The operation went well. There were no problems.

In anticipation of her return to high school in September, Adriana received her DTP booster (Repevax) on July 16, 2010. In retrospect, we think this vaccine only worsened the effects of her Gardasil injections.

On the 23rd of July 2010, one week after her DTP booster, we left for two weeks on holiday with our eldest daughter and Adriana. Though very cheerful at first, Adriana's behavior gradually changed. She became reserved, almost as if she were absent. She even talked about wanting to return home. We put it on record as getting a 'little blue' because she was far from her boyfriend.

The first week of our holiday went pretty well except that she always looked tired. She had no appetite and lacked enthusiasm. Nevertheless, she still participated in activities, walks, visits and games. It was during the second week that other disorders began to rear their ugly head. Now, in addition to all of the other mysterious symptoms Adriana was dealing with she began to be quite forgetful, experience more anxiety attacks and fears, moments of aggression which she quickly regretted, and losing her bearings. We consulted a general practitioner in the community. He put her symptoms down to mild depression and prescribed an anti-depressant to relax her. The day before our departure, our daughter had not improved so we went back to see what should be done. He told us to continue her medication and consult her regular GP when we got home.

On August 7, 2010, we took to the road again to reach our home.

The following morning, Adriana alternated between being agitated and calm. She was having difficulty walking. We immediately took her to the emergency room of the nearest hospital. By the time we arrived, she could not stand on her legs and looked completely lost.

This is where the nightmare began. Adriana was bombarded with questions from the emergency room doctor while she was in a state that did not allow her to answer. He wanted to know if she had taken drugs in addition to what seemed like an endless stream of other questions. He asked everything in a rather lively tone, which had the effect of overwhelming her to the point where she no longer spoke.

The doctor did not want to hear anything when my wife tried to explain the situation or tried to answer his questions.

We were later shocked when we were asked to drive Adriana ourselves to a psychiatric hospital in the area while she was in such a state of absolute suffering. It seemed we had no option but to comply. Adriana was admitted to the psychiatric facility.

This was the last time we saw Adriana 'alive'. Visits were forbidden at the psychiatric facility 'until further notice'. It was a full week before we were allowed to see our daughter at a hospital in Toulouse where she had been urgently admitted. She was in an artificially induced medical coma with irreversible convulsions. She never left the hospital.

As her parents, we had always believed Adriana was suffering from a lot more than a so-called depressive state. The emergency room doctors never listened to us. The fact that she consulted a psychiatrist was enough to convince them to not investigate any further. They were content to refer her directly to a psychiatric hospital.

In our opinion, this condemned her to an environment which provided inadequate care, lack of proper medical examinations, inadequate medical care, and the unwarranted prescription of antipsychotic drugs. In short, we believe this was a complete waste of time leading to a fatal outcome.

In November 2011, we sent a letter to the neurologist who had followed our daughter's case to inform him of our suspicions about Gardasil. We sent a similar letter to another doctor from the same region who was also a politician. A response from this politician reached us at the end of January 2012. Attached to this response was a report from the AFFAPS (French Agency for Health Safety of Health Products) which refuted the involvement of Gardasil in the death of Adriana, invoking the claim that there was too long a delay between the vaccination and death. The report mentioned 'neuroleptic malignant syndrome' as a potential cause of death. (NMS is a life-threatening idiosyncratic reaction to antipsychotic drugs characterized by fever, altered mental status, muscle rigidity, and autonomic dysfunction.)

At the end of February 2012, we got an appointment with the Toulouse neurologist and informed him of the AFFAPS report, which did not satisfy us at all. We told him again about our suspicions regarding Gardasil. Upon our insistence, he promised to have the file reviewed by AFFAPS.

In June 2012, this specialist gave us a new report from AFFAPS. The words 'neuroleptic malignant syndrome' were no longer included. The College of Physicians was moving toward a diagnosis of autoimmune encephalitis. The new report stated that 'it was not possible under these conditions to exclude the Gardasil vaccine as a contributing factor in the occurrence of this adverse effect.'

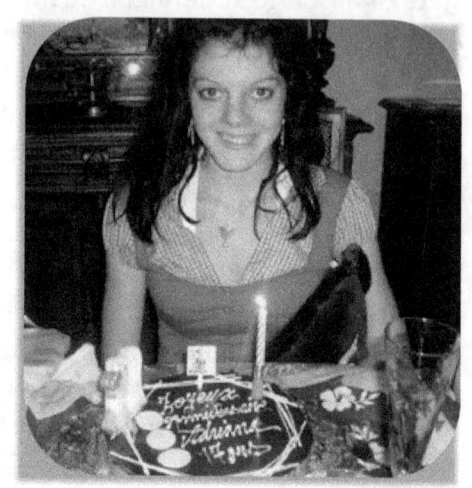

Early in 2014, on the advice of J. J. Bourguignon, we made contact with Mr. Coubris, an attorney in Bordeaux who was in charge of current Gardasil litigation. He helped us file a complaint against the laboratory Sanofi and AAFAPS.

We were summoned in September 2014 and again in December 2015 to appear before the Commission of Conciliation and Compensation (ICC) in Paris. These were particularly difficult events because we had to deal with people who have little regard for the victims.

When examining the voluminous medical records associated with Adriana's hospitalizations, the 'experts' limited themselves to bringing out only those elements tending to prove Adriana had psychological antecedents responsible for the eventual outcome. Her consultation with a psychiatrist was exploited from the beginning by all of the so-called 'expert witnesses'. They even went so far as to cite insignificant details from her public school records such as observations of her primary school teachers.

Their final conclusion was that in addition to psychological problems, Adriana had been unlucky enough to have contracted meningitis. Seriously??? They did not tell us when it could have occurred, which is strange to say the least when one considers the unsanitary conditions necessary for this disease to be transmitted. We point out that following the numerous examinations and tests which were performed during her hospitalizations, her doctors completely dismissed this hypothesis.

These experts even questioned the competence of the doctors from the University Hospital of Toulouse and AFFAPS who had acknowledged a possible accountability of Gardasil stating these specialists of province could not have fully read the post-mortem report prior to giving their opinion.

This 'conclusion' seems completely incomprehensible considering the fact that the post-mortem examination was conducted in the same hospital (the University Hospital of Toulouse) which was the recipient of the results of all tests performed by the doctors on their staff. Unfortunately, there were no representatives of this hospital present to deny the allegations put forth by the opposition or even to ask for the records to be checked.

We totally dispute the conclusion of the experts and the image they wanted to put forth regarding our daughter, who will always be remembered as being in good health before HPV vaccinations. The aim of the Commission was above all to eliminate Gardasil from any responsibility regarding our daughter's death.

They ignored our important question regarding the possibility of finding the presence of the aluminum adjuvant in post-mortem samples.

They did not discuss the medical deficiencies which occurred during Adriana's admission to the emergency room. They did not discuss the catastrophic hospitalization at the psychiatric hospital, including the fact that an electroencephalogram was conducted only after we insisted. They did not discuss the fact that the psychiatric facility did not provide for a daily reading of the EEG or the fact that it had to be interpreted four days later by a neurologist who was not on site. They did not discuss the fact that her EEG revealed severe cerebral dysfunction accompanied by suspected encephalitis. They did not discuss the fact that during the four days between when the EEG was done and the results were evaluated our daughter's condition became so critical that she required immediate transport to the University Hospital in Toulouse. They did not discuss whether her life could have been saved had she been transferred three days earlier.

Above all, they refused to discuss the fact that Adriana's EEG results confirmed she had a medical problem, NOT a psychological problem as we were told multiple times.

In November 2015, we were informed that the Paris prosecutor's office of criminal complaints had dismissed the Gardasil complaints. In this regard, it must be emphasized that no real investigation has been conducted. The situation has since stalled, but advertising for the new Gardasil is once again in the news.

We have always trusted medicine and vaccines. Today this is no longer the case.

Between our anger and immense sadness, we will continue to fight for our daughter and for all the victims the authorities refuse to acknowledge. We will continue to fight hoping that one day the scandal surrounding this poison vaccine will finally be revealed for all to see.

We are certain that the aluminum contained in Gardasil and DTP vaccines is responsible for our daughter's death.

Adriana was a dynamic and sporty girl, charming, smiling and quick-witted. She won the admiration of all. Adriana had a lot of plans. Unfortunately the cursed HPV vaccine shattered everything.

Norway

Gardasil had been approved in the United States under the condition that extensive follow-up studies be conducted in Norway which in practice meant that it would be necessary to include the vaccine in the children's vaccination program.

A contract was negotiated between FDA, Merck and the Norwegian government in 2006.[49] To date, the results of this study have not been accessible.

Norway began offering the HPV vaccine, Gardasil, to girls in the 7th grade (12-years-old) during the 2009/2010 school year as a part of the National Immunization Program. In 2016, Gardasil was also offered to women age 18 and up via a two-year catch-up program.[50]

In June 2015, Steinar Madsen, medical director of the Norwegian Medicines Agency reported they were investigating two cases where girls had symptoms 'that may be reminiscent of POTS.' At the time, the Norwegian Medicines Agency had received 581 reports of adverse reactions after Gardasil, 37 of them were classified as serious.[51]

Perhaps one of them was an 18-year-old girl whose report appeared in the news three months later. She had received all three injections of Gardasil during the first year of Norway's HPV vaccination program. After spending the next five years virtually bedridden, Maria finally received a formal medical diagnosis – POTS.[52]

According to the same article, POTS had been formally registered as a potential side-effect of Gardasil by the Norwegian Medicines Agency.

Somewhat ironically, over two decades before the introduction of Gardasil a group of scientists had decided to conduct a study to determine the prevalence of human papillomavirus in Norwegian

---

[49] June 8, 2006 Approval Letter – Human Papillomavirus Quadrivalent (Types 6, 11, 16, 18) Vaccine Recombinant; US FDA; accessed March 2019

[50] Staff writer; National surveillance of HPV vaccine programme; (NIPH) Norwegian Institute of Public Health; updated 24 Jan 2018; accessed March 2019

[51] Aase, K.A. and Stølan, Jorunn; HPV-vaccinated Norwegian girls are examined for new disease; Verdens Gang; 25 June 2015; accessed March 2019

[52] Stølan, Aarstad, Kristiansen; Took the HPV vaccine as a 12-year-old: Maria (18) has been seriously ill for five years; Verdens Gang; 21 Sept 2013, updated 21 Sept 2015; accessed March 2019

women who had been diagnosed with cervical cancer. From February of 1988 to April of 1989, the team collected biopsy samples from all women admitted to Norwegian Radium Hospital for the treatment of cervical cancer. Of all cancer samples analyzed, only 68% had HPV present.[53] The results of this study were published in January of 1994, fifteen years before the introduction of Gardasil into Norway's National Immunization Programme.

This study begs the question, "Why did Norwegian health officials recommend HPV vaccines as a cancer prevention measure when only 68% of their country's cervical cancer specimens showed the presence of HPV?" Were HPV vaccines truly worth the investment?

Beginning in the fall of 2018, Norway began offering Gardasil to boys as a part of the National Immunization Programme. One has to wonder how this expanded use was justified. Do the citizens of Norway have an unlimited healthcare budget?

---

[53] Kristiansen EWY, Jenkins, Andrew, Kristensen, Gunnar, Ask, Eirik, KaeRn, Janne, Abeler, Vera, Lindqvist, BJØRN H., TropE, Claes, Kristiansen, B.; Human papillomavirus infection in Norwegian women with cervical cancer; J. APMIS; January 1994; accessed March 2019

Never Give Up!

By Maria Lysaker Wennersberg, Rita Lysaker and Ranveig Brandsrud Henning, Mysen, Norway

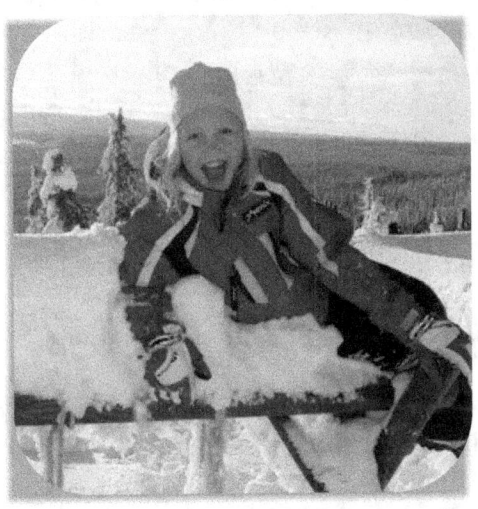

My name is Maria. I was born in 1997. In April 2018 I had my 21st birthday. For more than seven years I've been so ill I was not able to complete my junior school or high school education.

Before 2010 I was healthy and had a full social life with a wide circle of friends. I loved to be active and to compete. My favourite sports were skiing, football and handball. I had a good appetite and ate the same meals as the rest of the family – without problems. The only time I was in contact with a hospital was to have my tonsils removed when I was eleven years old.

Mamma is a nurse and our family has loyally followed the children's vaccination schedule. The information which was given to the parents at the school meeting about the HPV vaccine convinced Mamma that it was necessary and safe. Naturally she wanted to protect me from cervical cancer.

So, during 2009 and 2010 I received three injections of Gardasil. After the first shot I reacted with swelling at the injection site immediately, had a stomach ache and felt unwell.

Immediately after the second injection I had pain in my chest and went to the doctor. A few days later I went there again because of a sore and painful throat.

During the summer of 2010, I remember feeling more and more pain in my hips, joints and stomach, without thinking that this had any connection to the vaccine. As it turned out, this was only the beginning of my suffering.

In January 2011, several of my classmates had diarrhoea and I did too. I was home from school with an intense stomach ache, nausea and vomiting. After a few days I tried to go to school but couldn't manage. Stomach aches and pain which spread to other parts of my body put an end to further schooling for me.

As time went on, I became more and more tired and exhausted and my pains were persistent. I became more and more sensitive to light and sounds. Foods which I had loved before tasted different and I had difficulty eating. I tried to change my diet, cutting out milk, sugar and flour, but didn't get better.

I was often in contact with my local doctor, the outpatient emergency room (ER) and the local hospital. Many tests were taken but they could not find the reason I was ill. All the tests were fine.

Many different diagnoses, but no treatment options

In December 2011, I was diagnosed with **ME** (myalgic encephalomyelitis) at Fredrikstad Hospital, Østfold. My local doctor applied for me for training at the Catosenter, and I stayed there twice. I met other young people there who had ME and our days were filled with discussions, training, lectures and social meetings.

Being a competitive girl, I wanted to manage all the training activities as well as possible. So I pushed myself and became very tired. When I went home after the last session at the Catosenter in 2014 my health had not improved.

There were more visits to my local doctor, emergency rooms, and several hospital admissions. In March 2014, I was given a diagnosis of **Irritable bowel syndrome** from the Fredrikstad hospital.

On my eighteenth birthday I fainted when I was at my grandmother's. During the next days I fainted many times and was driven by ambulance to the local hospital.

New tests and examinations were done during the spring and I was given a new diagnosis by a cardiologist at Fredrikstad hospital: **POTS**. The treatments recommended were cognitive therapy, physiotherapy and compression stockings.

In the summer of 2015, I was very ill. ME got me down completely and the episodes of fainting/syncope were frequent. I went to the physiotherapist several times but because of exhaustion, pain and fainting it was difficult to continue the training program. Luckily the physiotherapist was very understanding about my problems.

Regarding cognitive therapy – I had previous experience with this, because when I couldn't manage to continue at secondary school after being diagnosed with ME, experts from the municipality with knowledge about ME were contacted. Their focus was on cognitive therapy. This didn't help at all and I became even more exhausted.

I had more blood tests done by my local doctor, but they were always fine despite the fact I was becoming more and more ill and thinner and thinner.

During the spring of 2015, my cardiologist diagnosed me with **POTS** (postural orthostatic tachycardia syndrome). This was a condition we had never heard about. What was going on with my health?

Putting the pieces together

In the summer of 2015, we read an article in the newspaper "VG" about the HPV vaccine and side effects. So far, none of us had even considered that my HPV vaccinations might be connected to the unusual medical problems I was having. A condition called POTS was described, then the article went on to mention ME. Both were conditions I had been diagnosed with. Was it possible they were a side-effect of the HPV vaccines I had received?

After searching on the net, we found Dr. Jesper Mehlsen at Fredriksberg Hospital near Copenhagen. I got an appointment there in August. I travelled there with Mamma and my grandmother. I was in a wheelchair but I lay in the car for most of the journey.

Dr. Mehlsen believed in me. This was the first time that I felt I was understood. A new tilt test was done and the following was written in my medical report:

> *"Suspected side effects of HPV vaccination. Received the first vaccination in November 2009 and the last one in May 2010. Has been ill for 4 ½ years. Has headaches, dizziness, fatigue, muscle weakness, orthostatic intolerance, and hip pain. Bedridden most of the time. Unable to eat much. Feels cold. Paraesthesia. Medicines: None. Daily fluid consumption: less than one liter. Extreme tachycardia which prevents the patient from*

standing and walking. Significant improvement of intravenous rehydration. It is suggested that rehydration is given in the same way by the doctor in Norway and that this should be combined with gradual activation in a standing position so that natural rehydration will occur. Calorie rich fluids are recommended for a while as the patient is presently undernourished and probably cannot be physically active to much extent for this reason. The patient's local doctor in Norway may contact the undersigned."

After returning to Norway I immediately contacted my local doctor with the papers from Dr. Mehlsen. Unfortunately, there was no willingness to give me intravenous saline treatment which was recommended by Dr. Mehlsen. According to medical experts at the local hospital and the ME center at the hospital in Oslo intravenous fluid therapy was not an approved treatment and no one would take responsibility for administration of intravenous saline.

The treatment which my local physicians recommended was again: cognitive therapy, gradual training and compression stockings, and that I should drink plenty of fluids.

As my condition developed, I became more and more exhausted, thinner and thinner but I tried to keep my courage up.

My POTS doctor at Fredrikstad hospital had promised me an appointment in September 2015 for a new examination, but because I hadn't followed her advice about treatment I was not given an appointment.

I explained to my local doctor that I was too ill to cope with the recommended treatment but that I wanted to have the appointment for a new examination.

I was finally given the appointment and I managed the meeting with the cardiologist and a new doctor. The new doctor promised me that he would contact Dr. Mehlsen. He also said he would find out if I could have the intravenous saline treatment at the Østfold hospital.

Quite optimistic, I went with Mamma and my great-aunt for this appointment. But unfortunately nothing happened after that. Mamma tried to make contact with both doctors several times. I wanted to know what Dr. Mehlsen said about intravenous treatment and whether the hospital leaders had approved it.

It felt as though everyone was deaf, I was not seen or understood, and so all doors were closed. I felt I had the right to an answer about the promise which was made at the meeting and I complained to the Health and Social Services Ombudsman in Østfold, but I didn't get any support from there either.

Meanwhile, I was getting more and more ill. Contact with the ambulance team and ER were more and more frequent – because of ME and because of losing consciousness/syncope and POTS.

The stomach pain was chronic, so were my headaches, nausea, vomiting, blurred vision, internal shivering and minor cramps which after a while became more intense and persistent. The extreme pain

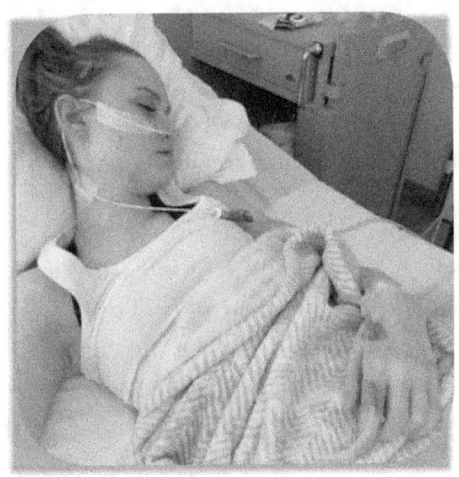

lead to unconsciousness, also seizures which could last for several hours.

In spring, 2016 I was again admitted to Kalnes hospital neurology department as an emergency case – with chronic pain, seizures and because of losing consciousness.

I asked for help for the pain many times. I wanted to have contact with the hospital's special pain team but I was refused each time.

It surprised me that as soon as I was admitted to Kalnes hospital I was given intravenous saline treatment. Why didn't they do this before – in August 2015 – when Dr. Mehlsen recommended it? Could some of my problems have been avoided if my fluid balance had been better many months earlier?

At the hospital I mentioned Dr. Mehlsen's and my suspicions – that my suffering from ME and POTS may be due to the HPV vaccine, but they wouldn't listen. They did many more tests but didn't suggest any treatment. All the test results were fine.

After several weeks at Kalnes, I was transferred to the neurology department at Rikshospital in Oslo. There too, intravenous treatment was started from the first day, but there was no interest in listening to me when I mentioned the HPV vaccine and Dr. Mehlsen's assumptions and medical report.

They did many tests, but all results were normal even though I was undernourished and there was no improvement regarding my pain, nausea, vomiting or seizures. I was at the hospital for ten weeks, was subjected to very demanding tests and examinations and then was sent home with advice to contact the district psychiatric center.

What was I to think? The local hospital Kalnes and the main hospital in my district (Rikshospital) did not believe I was physically ill. Did they really think all of my ME pain, suffering, seizures, and syncope would disappear if I contacted a local psychiatrist?

What did I do? I went as often as I could manage to the district psychiatric center. I couldn't get there every time, but once I met an experienced psychiatrist – a very positive meeting. I felt that I was listened to and understood. He told me I was strong and he wished me luck. He had no plans for treatment, but his words gave me hope.

Looking for help outside the Norwegian Health Service again

When I was in hospital some of my ME friends told me about an ME clinic in Brussels, so we decided to try Belgium. Blood samples were taken and sent to the Dr. Hertoghe clinic, and with good help from my family and friends we made the long journey by car to the clinic.

The doctor there explained the results of the tests and was glad that I had managed the journey. She told me that I was very ill, but that I would recover. She said that my adrenal glands were not functioning as well as they should and that I had a high aluminium concentration in my body. I was diagnosed with **adrenal gland failure and aluminium poisoning.** She gave me a detailed treatment plan before I left for the return trip home.

Once back in Norway, I started taking the prescribed minerals, vitamins and hormones. After a while with this treatment plan I felt some improvement – a little less nausea, fewer fainting episodes and sleep became more normal.

I was still undernourished and the ME pains were still there. I was still struggling, but sometimes managed to have a little social life. However, every time I tried there was a big price to pay. A few hours out amongst friends resulted in many hours in bed with headache, stomach ache and exhaustion.

There were two more consultations in Brussels. The second one we travelled by plane with several members of my family. It was a huge strain, I lost consciousness whilst on the plane making an oxygen mask necessary. But we made it. My seizures became even more severe on this trip. I was admitted to the nearest hospital as an emergency case. Once there, the results of my blood tests were read, I was examined and a new treatment plan was made.

I couldn't manage to make the journey to Brussels for the third appointment in January 2018. Mamma and two others from the family went there to hear about the latest blood test results and get a plan for further treatment.

Which plan for treatment do I follow now in 2018? In the summer of 2017, I made contact with a private doctor in Oslo, Joakim Iversen. He has extensive knowledge about ME, metabolism and nutrition. He took my nutritional problems seriously. Within two years my weight loss was 26 kg/57 lbs, (from 67 kg/147 lbs. down to 41 kg/90 lbs.). He took blood tests which were different from those which were taken at Kalnes hospital and Rikshospitalet. I have followed his treatment plan as best as I could.

2018: My medical condition now?

ME, POTS, seizures, and spasms are part of my everyday life. I often contact the emergency number 113. With my last seizure I was transported by ambulance helicopter to Kalnes. I feel that I'm mostly listened to and believed, even though some doctors show lack of understanding and empathy. Sometimes there are hurtful remarks.

My confidence in the local hospital has become far less during these years when I have been ill. Even though the leader of the team for pain treatment knows about my case, he has no suggestions for treatment of my cramps, seizures or chronic pains. Nobody knows how to relieve me of my pain or to stop my spasms and seizures.

In May 2018 I was acutely admitted to Kalnes hospital. The neurologist diagnosed me with **PNES (Psychogenic non-epileptic seizures).** His suggestion for treatment in my journal was:

> "Admission to the specialist hospital for epilepsy (SSE) for evaluation of PNES, further treatment locally, (in my opinion psychiatric)."

I have been referred to the specialist hospital for several examinations (stomach and seizures) but have been too ill to make the journey.

This autumn I managed to have an ECG test at a local hospital six miles from home. My local doctor arranged for an ambulance there and back. I have a good local doctor now who understands me and tries to help me. She visits me at home at least once a month.

I'm no longer undernourished, even though eating is still difficult. My stomach swells and I have intense stomach aches when I try to eat a little. I haven't used much energy lately as I can just about move from the bedroom to the sofa. I'm still struggling with nausea and violent vomiting.

Dr. Iversen has advised me to drink plenty of fluids, especially volvic water which can help the body to get rid of the aluminium from the vaccine. I sometimes vomit several liters of fluid. It makes me weaker and I feel frustrated that my body can't retain the fluids which I drink.

Since 2017 I have had a PICC line, and I'm glad about that. I get intravenous treatment at home at regular intervals.

Will I receive compensation for my vaccine injuries? My application to the Norwegian System of Patient Injury Compensation (NPE) was forwarded to an expert for an evaluation. I have been informed that the expert who is responsible for writing the evaluation has close connections with the vaccine industry, so my possibility for compensation will probably be minimal.

My everyday life now?

The chronic pain is there more or less all the time: headache, dizziness, numbness, hip pain, muscular pain, nausea, diarrhoea, vomiting, sometimes extremely hungry, other times no appetite, shivering, cold legs, concentration difficulties. The cramps start in the right thigh and after a couple of minutes develop into violent movements and I have intense pain in my whole body.

I often faint and float in and out of consciousness, whilst I hear that Mamma – my good helper – is there all the time asking me to breathe properly, measuring my pulse, temperature and oxygen saturation whilst she talks to emergency on 113 at the same time.

Needless to say, the situation is incredibly hard for Mamma and it is extremely tiring as she also has the rest of the family with children to care for.

Lately I've had seizures round about every third week and they sometimes last for several hours.

Mamma does an enormous job as my 'private nurse'. I need a lot, and get a lot of help from my close family. Throughout all these years Mamma, my stepsisters, grandmother, grandfather and the rest of my dear family have tried hard to help me. My great-aunt has a heart of gold and helps in every possible way. Without her support Mamma and I simply wouldn't be able to keep going.

My whole family is full of courage and optimism, turning lights on in the tunnels which come into in my life.

Of course I have dark days, hopeless days when the pain and suffering dominate. I've been out with friends twice since June 2018 and have paid dearly for it both times.

For the past year I've lived in my own flat and have got a dog called Hugo. I love my flat, but need a lot of help to be able to live here. For a short time I managed to take Hugo for a walk, but it has been several months since I could do it.

I have contact with Mamma by text messages and Snap on my telephone, but I have more difficulty now in concentrating and writing properly. Sometimes my messages are almost impossible to understand.

I have an alarm which I can press, so Mamma, grandmother and grandfather are warned quickly, but Mamma knows me so well that she appears when I need help – whether it's when I can't shower myself, have fainted or when the cramps have begun.

As it is now, I can't manage without Mamma, but I hope that this situation will change. She organises the PICC line, makes sure I take the right medicines, diet supplements and minerals which Dr. Iversen has prescribed. She buys everything that I need and helps with all my correspondence and appointments.

Mamma is the one who arranges that I have new blood tests taken which are sent to the doctors. The blood samples are drawn at my flat because I use so much energy to get to the lab several miles away. Mamma telephones and makes appointments so that those who do the blood sampling come at a time when it's not too difficult for me. I get very tired when there's fuss, stress, loud sounds and strong light. I'm also very restless when people who I don't know are around.

In October 2018, two new ladies came from the public administration department to find out what kind of help I needed. They were very nice and I think that I managed to explain my needs, even though I felt drained after they left.

The next few days I felt completely knocked out.

It has been a big strain for me that Mamma, who has been on sick leave for a long time, was dismissed this summer from her position as nurse in Eidsberg municipality. I know that if I hadn't been so ill Mamma would of course still have her job.

I hope that the ladies from the public administration department realize that I need help from a nurse and a lot of practical support - and that they find out about which steps should be taken to help me to get well and not more ill.

My dreams and wishes for the future

I dream about a life outside the flat, and nice walks in the fresh air with my dog Hugo.

I want to contribute actively and to spread information about my 'enemies' which are playing havoc with my body: ME, POTS, and all the other side-effects from the HPV vaccine.

I dream about freedom from the other enemies which belong to the medical establishment and are ruining my life:

- Lack of knowledge about vaccine injuries
- Lack of knowledge about methods for treatments
- Lack of understanding about vaccine victims' situation

I want to give correct information about the vaccine so that girls and boys may make an informed choice after they have learned about potential side-effects.

I hope that there will be more research on ME and autoimmune conditions so that new methods for treatment can be developed and used.

Sometimes I see myself on a stage talking about my life with all my 'enemies' with me saying, **"We must never give up!"**

Spain

HPV vaccination programs in Spain vary from one region to the next. Spain has nineteen regions, each responsible for determining and implementing their own healthcare policies and procedures. The Inter-Territorial Council of the National Health System acts as a coordinating body for all of Spain's autonomous regions. In 2007, the Inter-Territorial Council issued a recommendation for implementation of 3-dose HPV vaccination programs using either Gardasil or Cervarix throughout Spain targeting girls, age 11 to 14, with a preference for beginning at age 14. The recommended deadline for implementation was 2010. Three regions implemented programs in 2007, with the rest of Spain's regions beginning programs in the fall of 2008.[54]

On the 4th and 6th of February 2009, two girls were admitted to the same hospital in Valencia, both in critical condition after HPV vaccine administration. At the same time, a Majorcan girl was hospitalized with the same symptoms as the girls from Valencia. The Health Ministry issued a recall of 76,000 distributed doses of Gardasil batch number NH52670 after discovering the two girls from Valencia had both received injections from this batch.[55]

At first, the local Health Authorities in Valencia recognized a potential causal relationship between HPV vaccines and the convulsions of the girls. They seemed committed to discovering what happened. Despite having put their commitment in writing, meetings with Ministry of Health officials apparently changed their minds. No serious investigation was forthcoming.

---

[54] Supplement to: Bruni L, Diaz M, Barrionuevo-Rosas L, et al. Global estimates of human papillomavirus vaccination coverage by region and income level: a pooled analysis. Lancet Glob Health 2016; 4: e453–63. page 27, accessed March 2019

[55] Castillo, Raquel; Update 1-Spain halts batch of Merck's Gardasil; Reuters; 10 Feb 2009; accessed March 2019

9 July 2009, a petition for a Moratorium on HPV vaccine use was submitted to the Department of Health of the Valencian Community and the Spanish Ministry of Health. This petition was virtually ignored.

23 December 2009, the Ministry of Health received another petition with more than 9,500 signatures of people who wanted the health authorities to recognize the side effects girls suffered as a consequence of HPV vaccine use. Once again, there was no adequate response from the Ministry of Health.[56]

In January 2010, *Granada Today* published rather disturbing news for HPV vaccine stakeholders. The article reported that during the first year of their region's HPV vaccination program a full 58% of the 4600 eligible girls in their region had completed the three-dose series of HPV vaccines. The following year, 2009, only 31% finished the series. By 2010, only 6.8% of eligible girls completed the series despite the fact that the government offered Gardasil free of charge.[57]

In 2014, the Inter-Territorial Council of the National Health System recommended switching from the three-dose HPV vaccination to a two-dose schedule. By fall of the same year, most of Spain's autonomous regions had adopted the change.[58]

June 2014, a criminal complaint was filed against Merck-Sanofi Pasteur Laboratories, the Spanish National Health authorities and the regional health authorities of the La Rioja province alleging:

- fraudulent marketing and/or administration of an inadequately tested vaccine;
- failure to inform the public about the potential risks of using Gardasil;
- clear infringement of the right to informed consent;
- ignoring new medical conditions in those who used Gardasil despite the similarity of their symptoms and the relatively short period of time between vaccine administration and the onset of symptoms;

---

[56] Capilla, Alicia; HPV Vaccines in Spain: What happened to 'first do no harm'?; SaneVax Inc.; 25 Oct 2013

[57] Staff writer; Only six out of every hundred 14-year-old girls were vaccinated for papilloma in 2010; Granada Today; 17 Jan 2011; accessed March 2019

[58] Supplement to: Bruni L, Diaz M, Barrionuevo-Rosas L, et al. Global estimates of human papillomavirus vaccination coverage by region and income level: a pooled analysis. Lancet Glob Health 2016; 4: e453–63. page 27

- ignoring established and new scientific evidence illustrating the potential harmful effects of Gardasil ingredients and manufacturing methods;
- callous disregard for those suffering new medical conditions post-Gardasil;
- failure to inform the public that HPV infections are simply one of the risk factors involved in the development of cervical cancer;
- failure to inform the public that 90% of all HPV infections clear on their own without medical intervention;
- failure to inform the public about alternative methods of controlling cervical cancer; and
- criminal liability for the injuries resulting from the administration of Gardasil[59]

The following month, another high-profile complaint was filed on behalf one of the girls from Valencia who had become seriously ill after Gardasil injections. The allegations put forth were similar to those listed above with a strong emphasis on the alleged violation of the fundamental right to informed consent prior to any medical intervention.[60]

A few weeks later, representatives of AAVP (Association of People Affected by HPV Vaccines) met with Spanish Health Ministry officials to request the withdrawal of HPV vaccines from the national vaccination schedule of Spain because of the unusually high rate of serious adverse reactions and deaths reported not only in Spain, but around the world.[61] Evidently, their request fell on deaf ears. No one with enough power to change the national vaccination schedule wanted to address the unintended consequences of their nations' HPV vaccination program.

Meanwhile, Professor of Public Health at the *University of Alicante*, Dr. Carlos Alvarez-Dardet - a past president of the *European Public Health Association* and the *Spanish Society of Public Health and Health Administration*, launched a petition against HPV vaccines citing various

---

[59] Erickson, Norma; Gardasil: Criminal complaint filed in Spain; SaneVax Inc.; 2 Aug 2014

[60] Sarich, Christina; First HPV Vaccine Lawsuit Filed in Spain Against Manufacturers and Health Authorities; Natural Society; 23 July 2014; accessed March 2019

[61] Capilla, Alicia; AAVP ASKS Spanish Health Ministry to Ban HPV Vaccines; SaneVax Inc.; 29 Aug 2014

side effects occurring in girls after HPV vaccination including death, permanent disability due to nervous system disease, autoimmune disorders, pulmonary embolisms, Guillain-Barré syndrome, seizures, fainting, tremors, syncope, dizziness, pancreatitis, lupus, and others.

Alvarez-Dardet was also unhappy with the efficacy of the vaccine, claiming that it only protects against a few strains of HPV and this protection is short lived.

Dr. Carlos Alvarez-Dardet went so far as to state the vaccine is, "*not necessary or effective, and it's not even safe.*"[62]

By December 2015, his petition had over 35,000 signatures. Health officials were still not inclined to alter their recommendations for HPV vaccine use.

April 2017, the High Court of Justice of Asturias-Spain (TSJA) condemned the Asturian Health System for the death of Andrea, a young Spanish girl who died shortly after receiving the second injection of HPV vaccine.

This was a young woman with a medical history of mild episodes of bronchial asthma. When she got the first shot of HPV vaccine on July 23, 2012, she experienced a headache and severe exacerbation of her previously diagnosed asthma. Despite these warning signs, the second injection was administered on August 23, 2012. She immediately experienced severe difficulty breathing. When seizures began 12 hours later, she was moved to the Maternal and Child Hospital of the HUCA. She remained in the Pediatric Intensive Care Unit until she died on September 8th.

The judge ruled there was a causal association between the HPV vaccine and this young girl's untimely death. He also condemned the local health authorities for not recognizing her adverse response to the first injection and administering the second dose anyway.[63]

Spanish health officials have still not been moved to change their recommendations.

---

[62] Staff writer; Concerns Raised About HPV Vaccine; Healthplan Magazine; 3 Dec 2015; accessed March 2019

[63] Capilla, Alicia; HPV Vaccine: Death in Spain; SaneVax Inc.; 16 April 2017

Devastated and Deserted after Cervarix

By Marina from Spain

Hello, my name is Marina, I am one of the many girls affected by the Human Papillomavirus vaccine, Cervarix.

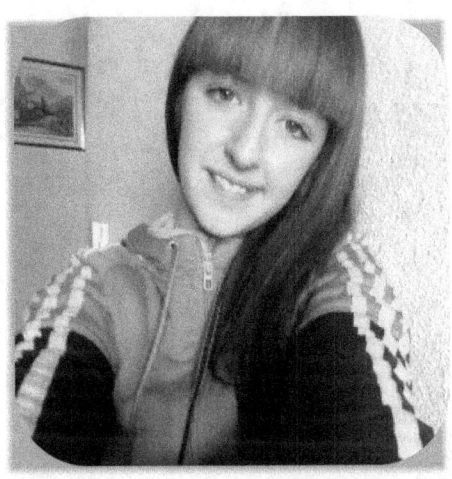

Once I was a very athletic girl, I loved rhythmic gymnastics, dancing, going for walks, and studying. My daily life was very busy, because I combined my studies with different activities. I loved going to the country with my family and walking along country roads, watching the almond trees bloom, the sunsets. In short, I led a normal life.

But all of this changed when I least expected it. I was on top of the world. I had no idea how drastically my life would be altered.

It all began as a perfectly normal day, I had class and I was walking to the institute. I liked to clear my head before going to class. I had no idea this would turn out to be the worst day of my life.

This was the day I was scheduled to get my first injection of Cervarix. I had no idea what would happen to me from that moment on.

Immediately after the shot I started to feel bad. I was unconscious in class and the teacher took me to my mother's work. We thought it was from having seen the needle. I wish it had been that simple. I only remember that my mother gave me an Ibuprofen and I went home to lie down because I was feeling very bad. When I woke up I was literally jumping on my bed, because of the tonic-clonic movements produced by an adverse effect of the vaccine, something that some doctors would not recognize as a potential side effect even though it is listed in the package insert. The one thing I did not expect was that a doctor would call me crazy that day.

In addition, I could not stop having seizures, no matter what medication they gave me, I just kept having seizures.

I ended up spending many days in the emergency room. After a multitude of tests, the final diagnosis was that everything was psychological. I knew this would be a problem, but I had no idea how big the problem would become.

Over the next few years, I spent days, weeks, months, years going from hospital to hospital, submitting to multiple really unpleasant tests, lumbar punctures, magnetic resonance images... all resulting in no

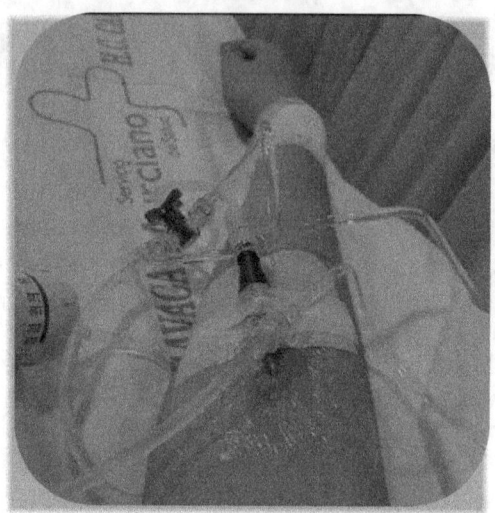

formal diagnosis. Because there was no formal diagnosis, psychosis was assumed.

I was unable to walk, suffering tremors and seizures. I lost control of my sphincter muscles. I had to go to class in a wheelchair to sit for my exams. I prepared for my exams on my own in the hospital. It was not fun, especially when I had symptoms of vertigo.

We were desperate. Nothing was normal any more. We had nowhere to turn.

We heard there was a doctor in Madrid who gave natural treatments and that several girls had improved under his care. So, we went there. Of course the trips from Murcia to Madrid were not very short. Although it was a slow and very expensive treatment, I improved a lot. The public health system covered none of the costs because supposedly all of my symptoms were of psychological origin.

There were only a few doctors who believed my health problems were medical. Thanks to them I had hope.

I would like to mention Dr. José María Melgares de Aguilar, he was great support for me and a great doctor. I saw him and he seemed like my salvation! Also Dr. Blas González Pina, an internist at the hospital in Caravaca de la Cruz (Murcia) where I reside. Due to their care, I have not had more crisis in a long time. I hope to continue like this.

After my Cervarix injection, I spent four years of my life in a wheelchair. This caused a great amount of suffering for me during what should have been some of the happiest years of my life.

The only thing I ask is that no more girls get vaccinated without knowing all of the facts. I feel the national health system has simply abandoned me and all the other girls like me.

I want no other girls to go through the same life-changing events I have had to experience.

My Cervarix Nightmare

By Patricia González, Spain

My name is Patricia González, I am 44 years old and I am one of many of the women affected by HPV vaccines in Spain.

I write these lines, to describe the horror and suffering that I have put up with and still endure after being vaccinated with Cervarix.

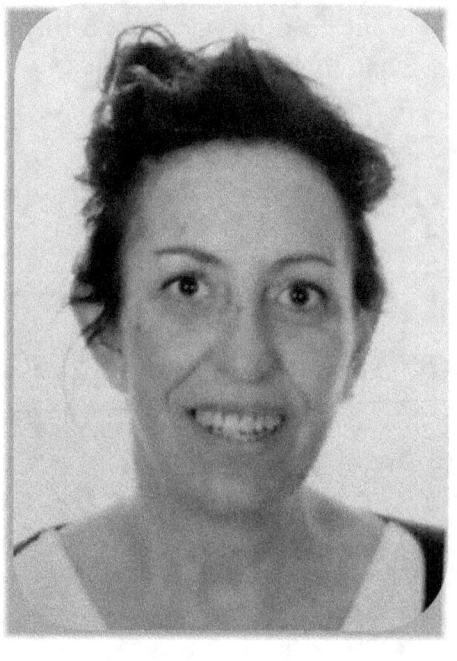

My nightmare started with a routine visit to the gynecologist at the age of 40. They told me that I had papillomavirus in the cervix. For that reason, I had biopsies every six months to control the infection. During the last scheduled appointment, in June 2017, cancer cells were found near the papillomavirus infection site. I got the results on August 5th and by the 25th of the same month I was in the operating room. The surgery went well, and the postoperative period was without complications.

During my next appointment, the gynecologist suggested, actually it was more of a command for me to have the controversial HPV vaccine. I refused and the doctor became very angry and told me that with the family history I had, the vaccine would give me antibodies, and so on... At no time did I sign any informed consent papers and I was not told about the possible adverse reactions I could suffer. I had serious doubts about vaccinating myself because for me that year 2017 was a very peculiar year in relation to family matters. Finally, I decided to get the vaccine.

I got the first shot on 5th January 2018, afterwards my arm swelled but I did not pay much attention to that.

The real nightmare started when I got the second shot on February 5th, two days after I thought I was dying due to the headaches. They were horrible. I was still working but I had to take some time off sick, as they were unbearable. I visited emergency rooms 15 times or more. I frequently needed oxygen, valium and calming medicine intravenously and then they sent me back home. Nobody thought to send me to the neurologist. Finally it was my family GP who asked for a quick appointment with the neurologist.

During the appointment with the neurologist I explained I was suffering these pounding headaches since I got the second shot of the HPV vaccine and that I had never had such migraines before. It took a month to find the right drug/medicine that I should take for my pounding headaches. The migraines disappeared, but the nightmare continued as I started having attacks that at first seemed epileptic but without loss of consciousness. I had the first crisis while I was working.

In addition, I started having seizures and sphincter loss. I was admitted to the hospital. The nightmare had started again: neurological tests, repeated crisis, 15 times to hospital... doctors make reference to the vaccine, but they do not certify anything in writing.

I have seen multiple psychiatrists, psychologists, who discharged me from hospital because they did not find anything strange in my behavior.

My life has changed completely. I cannot go alone on public means of transport, and I cannot have a normal life such as going to the cinema or hanging out with my friends, because of the crisis.

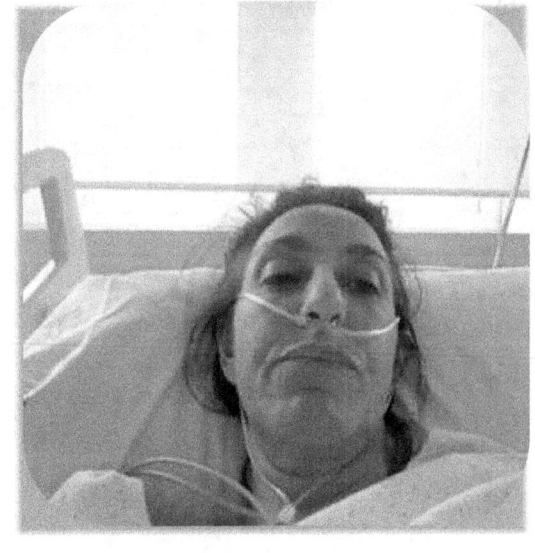

Finally, the doctors diagnosed pseudo crisis. There are no medicines for this, only valium and going to the hospital. This has been my life since June.

Now, thankfully I am being treated by a Naturist doctor. I am feeling much better, because he is doing liver and kidney cleanses. What annoys me most about all of this is I am personally paying for private doctors. The National Health Service has nothing to offer because they cannot classify my disease and for that reason I am placed in the rare diseases category. This basically means I am on my own for treatment options. I´ve seen all sorts of specialists.

That is what has happened to me in relation to the neurologic problems I am suffering. But this is not all, I am also suffering from gynecological problems. I have lost my period. Doctors wanted to diagnose me with ovarian failure. I asked them to test my hormone levels. It was discovered that I am neither menopausal nor peri-menopausal. I am simply not menstruating, apparently as a consequence of the vaccine. On top of that, now I have a cyst in the ovary that I have to get rid of.

I had visited the gynecologist on seven occasions, and each time a different gynecologist has seen me. And of course, each one has given me a different diagnosis. However nobody has read my medical history. On one of the visits they prescribed me some tablets. During the last visit they took them away because I had a high risk of having a stroke.

My life has been destroyed. I cannot go anywhere alone for fear I will have another medical crisis. I have been off work sick since February 2018. I have no idea whether my life will ever be normal again.

I want to thank the Association of the Affected People in Spain (AAVP), for the support which they have given to me at all times and their desire to fight for HPV vaccine survivors like me.

The United Kingdom

Due to the implementation of a national cervical cancer screening program, the mortality rate for cervical cancer fell nearly 60% in the United Kingdom between 1974 and 2004.

JCVI (Joint Committee on Vaccines and Immunizations) is a standing committee charged with providing impartial advice to the Secretaries of State for England, Scotland, Wales and Northern Ireland. In 2005, the JCVI was informed of the development of two HPV vaccines, Cervarix and Gardasil, which may aid in efforts to control cervical cancer.

After reviewing HPV vaccines no less than seven separate times, the JCVI recommended instituting a national immunization program for girls age 12-13 throughout the United Kingdom in early 2008. The committee also recommended a catch-up program for girls from age 14-18 for a limited time.[64]

Additional recommendations of JCVI included a statement that HPV vaccination of those who were pregnant should be deferred until after the pregnancy. The committee also determined that vaccinations of females over the age of 18 and vaccination of males was not a cost effective option according to the information available at the time.

The decision of which HPV vaccine to choose was left open to price negotiation. Ultimately, the UK chose to introduce routine HPV vaccinations with Cervarix.

According to an article by investigative journalist Christina England, just hours before the new HPV vaccination program was formally announced, a promotional DVD was sent to every General Practitioner (GP) in the United Kingdom. She stated:

"The DVD was posted with the G.P. magazine and was a clever marketing strategy aimed at busy G.P.'s to 'brainwash' them into

---

[64] JCVI; Statement on Human Papillomavirus vaccines to protect against cervical cancer; UK government; accessed March 2019

believing that the Cervarix vaccine protected young women from the perils of cervical cancer. With phrases such as 'Cervarix, the vaccination to prevent cervical cancer' and convincing animation, the DVD certainly goes all out to convince the medical profession that the vaccine is safe, effective, and a must for all young women."[65]

During 2008-09, the National Health Service sponsored an advertising campaign with the slogan "Armed for Life." This campaign represented an investment of £2.8 million to promote the new HPV vaccination program.[66]

By September 2009, there had been over 2,000 reports of adverse reactions recorded in the UK after Cervarix vaccinations. An analysis conducted by the Medicines and Health care products Regulatory Agency (MHRA) revealed 2,107 patients reporting, with several reporting multiple reactions for a total of 4,602 suspected side-effects. These reactions included teens suffering convulsions, eye rolling, muscle spasms, seizures and hyperventilation soon after Cervarix administration.[67]

February 2010, investigative journalist Christina England wrote an article protesting the NHS sponsored 'Armed for Life' campaign claiming the advertisements were untrue and should be banned. She was referring to advertisements plastered on the sides of buses used for transportation along every school route in West Sussex and the route to a local hospital. The advertisements proclaiming Cervarix would ensure you were 'armed for life' against cervical cancer were also posted inside the buses and on bathroom doors in local cinemas.

According to Christina, and multiple scientists around the world, giving medical consumers the impression of lifelong protection from the possibility of contracting cervical cancer was an out and out lie. Christina felt compelled to file a formal complaint with the Advertising Standards Authority (ASA).

Evidently, ASA agreed. On 3 March 2010, they issued a notice that the situation had been resolved informally. The Advertising Standards

---

[65] England, Christina; GlaxoSmithKline Brainwashed Doctors about HPV Vaccine; 2 Nov 2010; accessed March 2019

[66] Filby, Grace; Truth about Cervarix; Grace Filby's Pigeon Post; accessed March 2019

[67] Donelly, Laura, Health Correspondent; Two thousand schoolgirls suffer suspected ill-effects from cervical cancer vaccine; The Telegraph; 12 Sept 2009; accessed March 2019

Authority ordered the words 'arm yourself for life' be changed or removed from all advertising. Subsequently, the UK Department of Health advertising campaign was halted and all references to 'armed for life' removed from government sponsored websites.[68]

In October 2010, two primary care trusts teamed up to offer 'Love to Shop' vouchers to girls ages 16 to 18 provided they showed up for all three injections of Cervarix. If a girl submitted to all three injections, she would receive £45 worth of vouchers she could spend at various high-end stores.[69]

By November 2010, after 75 potential adverse reactions to Cervarix had been reported in Scotland, the government moved to reassure the public that the HPV vaccine was safe. The Scottish government's reassurances basically fell into three categories. 1) Adverse event reports filed after Cervarix injections do not necessarily mean the vaccine caused the new medical condition. 2) There is no proven link between Cervarix and adverse events. 3) The HPV vaccine is safe – clinical trials and close monitoring by MHRA have proven this.[70]

2010, the UK instituted a new law called 'The Bribery Act.' This law bars any company operating in Britain, whether foreign or domestic, from making an illicit payment to public officials, private citizens, or businesses. According to *The Wall Street Journal,* British officials may use the law to target pharmaceutical companies.[71] This law was scheduled to take effect in April 2011.

In a press release issued by the Department of Health and Social Care on 24 November 2011, Professor David Salisbury, the government's Director of Immunization, announced that beginning in September of 2012 the HPV vaccine of choice in the UK would be Gardasil. According to Professor Salisbury, it was not unusual to change vaccines following competitive tendering exercises, or when new research findings come to light. The press release did not mention

---

[68] Staff Writer; Cervarix-Armed for Life? United Kingdom says 'NO' as they battle false advertising; SaneVax Inc.; 6 Jan 2011

[69] Martin, Danial; HPV voucher bribe for teenage girls to have cervical jabs; Fury at 'promiscuity scheme' as NHS faces cuts; The Daily Mail; 26 Oct 2010; accessed March 2019

[70] Aitken, Mark; Cervical cancer jabs are still safe for girls insists Scottish Government; The Daily Record; 14 Nov 2010; accessed March 2019

[71]Corcoran, Patrick; British Bribery Law Worries U.S. Drug Companies; FairWarning.org; 28 Dec 2010; accessed March 2019

which of these circumstances prompted the decision to change from Cervarix to Gardasil. The HPV vaccine change did not affect the administration recommendations, or the recommendation that HPV vaccinations be carried out in school-based settings to facilitate maximum uptake. The final line of the press release stated, "Vaccination is voluntary, not mandatory."[72]

In spite of the fact health authorities insisted HPV vaccines were safe, a health watchdog admitted over a thousand reports of suspected side-effects had been filed during the first six months of the Gardasil campaign. According to the March 2013 article, reports included cases of 12 and 13-year-old girls with seizures, breathing difficulties, joint pain, fatigue and/or stomach problems.[73]

The JCVI announced that recent research showed antibody response to two doses of HPV vaccine for adolescent girls was as good as a three-dose regime. Therefore, beginning in March of 2014 the UK would join Switzerland, The Netherlands, Mexico, and Quebec by recommending a change to a two-dose schedule for girls who started the series when they were under age 15. This change took effect in September 2014, at the beginning of the academic year.[74]

August 2015, Freda Birrell addressed the Scottish Petitions Committee on behalf of over 200 UK Association for HPV Vaccine Injured Daughters (AHVID) along with over 2,000 people from 55 countries who were having similar issues and thus supported her request to urge the Scottish Government to convene a roundtable discussion on the safety of HPV vaccines with medical/scientific professionals from both sides of the debate.[75]

In an article published in *The Daily Mail,* September 2017, it was disclosed that Dr. Ian Hudson, MHRA chief executive had written to Richard Benyon the Conservative MP for Newbury, stating, "The fact that we have received more reports for HPV vaccine than other vaccines does not in itself raise any particular concerns."[76]

---

[72] Department of Health and Social Care press release; HPV vaccine to change in Sept 2012; 24 Nov 2011; accessed March 2019

[73] Boyle, Janet; UK: Concerns over cervical cancer jab side-effects; *The Sunday Poste;* 3 March 2013; available on SaneVax.org

[74] Ibid ref #63

[75] The Scottish Parliament; PE01574: HPV Vaccine Safety; Petitioner, Freda Birrell; 21 August 2015; accessed March 2019

[76] Tanner, Claudia and Deevay, Jacqui; Teenager died in her sleep weeks after

Evidently, the international controversy that existed did not make any difference to those charged with protecting the health and well-being of UK citizens. In July of 2018, public health minister Steve Brine announced England would join the Welsh and Scottish governments by offering the HPV vaccine to boys ages 12 to 13. Apparently, the JCVI issued a statement the week before indicating that a more 'gender-neutral' programme battle HPV infections would be 'cost-effective.'[77]

Needless to say, this decision left UK citizens wondering whether or not their health officials understood the term 'precautionary principle'.

being given HPV vaccine as experts reveal the lives of thousands of girls have been destroyed by the controversial jab; The Daily Mail; 27 Sept 2017, updated 6 Oct 2017; accessed March 2019

[77] Bulman, May; HPV vaccination to be introduced for all teenage boys in UK, government announces; The Independent; 24 July 2018; accessed March 2019

England

Challenged and Re-Challenged by HPV Vaccinations

By Phyllis Samuels, Stockton-on-Tees, Cleveland, UK

My daughter, Beth was an active energetic child. From age 4 she engaged in dance lessons at least three times per week enjoying ballet, tap, modern and jazz. She also loved acting and participated in stage school lessons each week. Beth performed at yearly charity shows and a local Stage Society Show at a thriving theatre. She loved her parts in *Annie, Oliver,* and

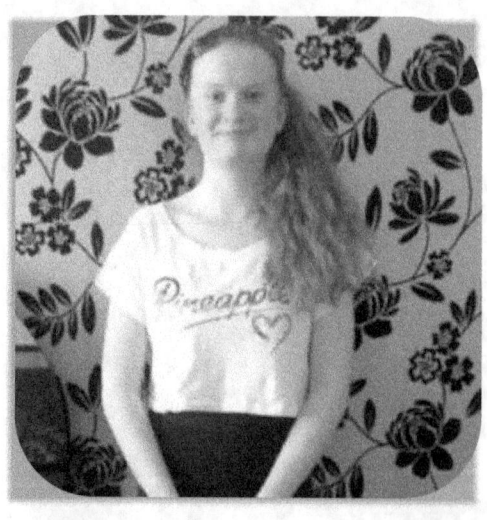

Pinocchio. Since the devastating impact of her HPV vaccinations, she is no longer able to dance; but she continues with her passion for acting. She has played roles in *Whistle Down the Wind, Calamity Jane* and is currently rehearsing for her role in *Chitty Chitty Bang Bang.*

She had a large circle of friends, loved school and was a grade A student. She enjoyed Brownies and Guides and being a Police Cadet with our local force helping others and learning about the role of the police.

She was able to partake in some very memorable activities including taking part in a reconstruction for a Crime and Investigation documentary. Probably even more memorable for her was having the privilege of walking out the Spanish Football Team at the World Cup Final in South Africa in 2010 as a Player Escort. Following a national competition one child was selected to represent each country. Beth had the honor of being selected as the representative for England. She loved the event and was able to meet people like Nelson Mandela.

Beth loved family holidays, shopping for clothes, spending time with her family and her many extra-curricular activities. She loved being a normal, happy, very active teen. All of that changed following her HPV vaccinations.

Why did we consent?

Beth lost her godmother to cancer and I have had cancer twice. With our history, the literature on HPV vaccination seemed very compelling. The information leaflet listed a limited number of potential adverse reactions limited primarily to inflammation and soreness at the injection site. With our family history, it seemed a no-brainer to proceed with the vaccinations. I will always regret this life-changing decision.

Beth had her first injection and within approximately 48 hours had a doctor's appointment because of a raging headache that radiated heat from the headache site. The GP referred her to a pediatrician to consider if any further investigation was required and specifically a brain tumor was ruled out.

Around the same time, Beth began experiencing severe abdominal pains. These were extensive and resulted in periods of hospital admission with suspected appendicitis. Consequently, she started to miss time at school due to ill health. This severely impacted both her friendships and education.

Blood tests had revealed a vitamin D deficiency so supplements were prescribed.

Beth's second injection was followed by additional problems. Initially, there was pain and swelling in her joints resulting in a referral to a consultant at a more specialized hospital to consider the prospect of arthritis diagnosis. Without any tests being done, the consultant ruled this out.

Beth's health continued to decline. She was now suffering constant periods of chronic fatigue. Her attendance at dancing and stage school declined as did her school attendance. She needed to rest or sleep constantly and was very lethargic. These conditions continue to this day.

Beth had new medical conditions after her first and second jabs, but the third injection was catastrophic. On the day of her third jab, she had PE at school and her legs simply gave way beneath her resulting in her falling to the floor. She was very sweaty, pale and clammy.

She became very weak and constantly continued to present with raging headaches, joint swelling and pain, abdominal difficulties, chronic fatigue etc. Over the weeks and months following her third vaccination, she continued to have pervasive weakness in her legs. She had to stop dancing as she would stumble when her legs gave way beneath her.

It was heart breaking for her and her family to watch her peers, friends with whom she had grown up compete in dance shows and exams.

She woke up one morning and told us she could not feel her feet. They were very cold to touch and had poor circulation. When we pressed a finger on her skin, it would remain white for a long period before the color returned. We took her to the local walk-in center via a piggyback. She was immediately admitted to the hospital. Over the course of the day, the loss of feeling increased moving up to her knees. So, the following day she was transferred to a more specialized hospital in Newcastle.

Over that weekend she lost all feeling from her waist down. She spent three months in hospital prior to a Christmas day break at home before returning to hospital for over three more months. During that time, despite daily physiotherapy together with hydrotherapy no improvements occurred. Her legs were always freezing cold. Very often blue and with limited circulation.

To this day, over three years later, she remains paralyzed from the waist down.

Recently she was an inpatient for a urine/ kidney infection. The treating doctor advised she had lost all of her muscle tone so would never be able to walk again. This is heart breaking.

Over the last three years, she has been diagnosed with various medical problems that continue to impact her daily life significantly. She has difficulties with her bladder, retains urine and as a result experiences a high number of infections. At times her body retains urine to the extent her stomach swells, bladder scans reveal dangerously high volumes of urine retention, so she is catheterized to remove it.

Her last hospital admission for this lasted 10 days, but this is a regular occurrence usually requiring IV antibiotics for one to two weeks to clear the infection.

Her bladder is regularly checked and now showing signs of an inability to cope with such issues. Her kidneys are starting to struggle also. She had a hospital admission in August/September with severe kidney pain and vomiting a thick black liquid.

At times she has profound difficulty swallowing which resulted in recent hospitalizations due to ulcers throughout her esophagus. The ulcers cause swelling so she is unable to eat, struggles to drink and required another 7-day admission to the hospital. She continues to have ulcers throughout her esophagus.

Her liver is damaged. Typically liver enzymes should be approximately 30-45. Beth's frequently are in excess of 100. Last week it was 176. She passes out or becomes very weak resulting in a real need to eat to get sugar for energy.

In November 2018, following one such episode she was admitted to the hospital and needed bags of IV glucose because of her very low blood sugar level. A common effect is she develops itchiness all over her body.

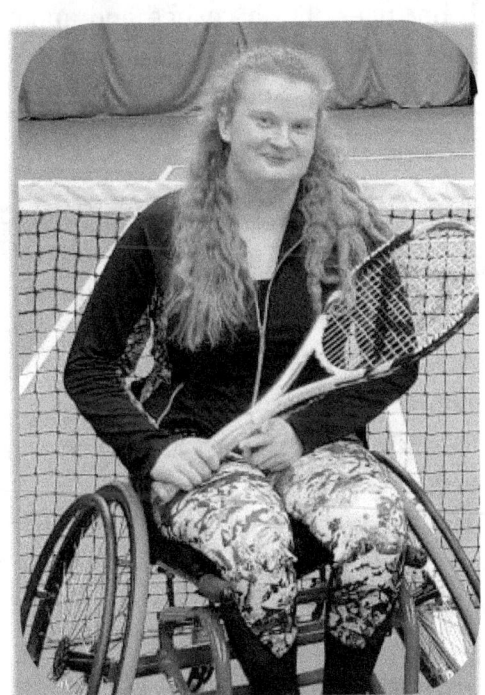

She always needs someone with her due to the unpredictability of her becoming weak and passing out. Her organs are really struggling.

Her bowels do not function correctly. She regularly has blood in her 5 to 6 bowel movements each day. This continues to be looked in to.

Beth has other difficulties such as losing the skin on her head, fingers and other parts of the body and her big toe nail grows in a way that has required one to be permanently removed. The other is constantly infected and causes her toe to bleed so is likely to need removing imminently.

The most recent difficulty that Beth has presented with is what appeared to be nodules on her finger. Following an ultra sound and MRI this has been diagnosed as a tumor which must be removed urgently as it is wrapped around her nerve sheath. It is growing rapidly and we have just been given Beth's date for surgery. The difficulties with this is being a wheel chair user Beth requires the use of her hands and fingers to transfer and wheel, so this will further compromise her independence and ability to get around.

Unusually from what I understand of such cases, there is now a recording in Beth's medical notes to confirm that Beth has had a sensitivity to the HPV vaccination and the reaction has been reported.

The impact on Beth has been catastrophic. Physically, every day is a struggle due to her competing health needs. She remains constantly exhausted.

Nothing can be planned as we cannot predict when her health will further deteriorate. She missed a significant amount of schooling and continues to do so. This has impacted her education, friendships, and ultimately her future.

It is heartbreaking to watch her peers finish college and apply for university. Beth has to sit by and watch her friends pass their driving tests, drive, and forge their own independent paths in society. She has to watch as they obtain part-time jobs, commence relationships and pursue their passions.

Meanwhile, due to her disabilities, her paralysis and complex medical needs, Beth struggles with every part of day-to-day life. I cannot begin to explain how hard this is for me, as her mother, to watch.

I have no idea what Beth's future holds. I would love for her to be independent and be able to follow her dreams. I would love to see her be free of pain and be able to follow in the footsteps of her peers, but I know these things will not happen.

More than anything I want her to be happy, to be able to live her life independently and reach her full potential, but given how regularly she experiences new medical problems, I fear further symptoms are lurking just around the corner.

Scotland

Functional Disorder, or Medical Issues?

By Caran Dynan, Kilsyth Scotland

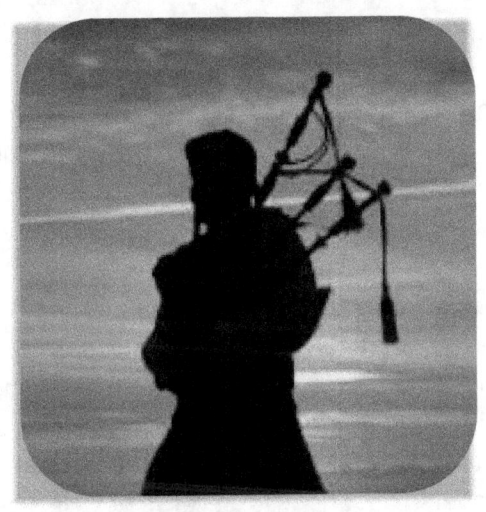

Amy was born perfectly healthy and grew up normally. She developed hay fever, something common in our family, but other than this she kept well.

Amy had a slight shyness but she was a very happy girl surrounded by loving family and had no problem making and keeping friends. By the time she went to school she made a number of friends both at school and at the afterschool group she attended.

Amy's biological father was never in the picture but I spoke openly and honestly to her about this. When she was 9 years old I met my current husband, who had a 6-year-old son. Amy got on brilliantly with my husband and still does. She also got on great with his son and within time looked on him as a little brother as well as a friend.

My husband and I had a son when Amy was almost 11 years old and she loved showing him off to her friends when I picked her up from school.

When she progressed to high school, she liked it for a while, keeping up a high standard of school work. She enjoyed spending time with friends, going out for walks with us as a family and generally just being a normal young girl.

She received the HPV Vaccine in October 2012, which is when things started to change.

Within a week of receiving the vaccine, Amy fainted, something she had never ever experienced before. This started to become quite a regular occurrence.

She also rapidly developed severe social anxiety and where she once had quite a large group of friends, she started to separate herself from them and avoided social situations.

She got to the point where she could no longer face school, trembling with tears at the thought of going. We could not understand what had happened to cause these sudden changes. We had several meetings with the school and talked extensively with Amy about the possibility of her being bullied as it was the only thing we could think of (at least for the social aspects, although it would not explain the fainting), she denied profusely that this was an issue. No staff member at the school had witnessed any bullying, including a guidance teacher who had been keeping a closer eye on Amy due to her own concerns over the sudden change in Amy.

When she did manage to attend school, she was set up with meetings with the school counsellor, again there was no mention or evidence of any bullying. Amy was having really dark thoughts about harming herself and worse. She was terrified of leaving the house. She found it increasingly difficult to speak to anyone, not only people she did not know, but family members too. She also became very lethargic and would sleep most of the day where possible.

Amy attended a few sessions with Child and Adolescent Mental Health Services, with myself and my parents. Amy found it easier in family sessions as she did not have to speak as much, but the sessions were emotionally draining. She felt like she could not give any 'useful' answers about why she felt so low and detached because she did not understand herself what was happening to make her feel like this. She decided she did not want to go to CAMHS anymore as she felt that no progress was being made and she dreaded the sessions.

We were referred back to CAMHS at a later date as the doctors advised that whatever Amy was experiencing stemmed from a psychological problem even though there were physical attributes such as weakness, fainting, constant headaches, irregular heartbeat, etc. Again, this was not helpful and we were advised there was not much they could do. In fact, we were actually accused by the counsellor of enabling Amy to feel the way she did.

Amy became so introverted she was unable to go into a shop and buy something herself or start any type of conversation with someone she was not very close to. She had changed so dramatically, there was a point that I thought she maybe had a condition called Selective Mutism or had even developed a form of Autism or Asperger's Syndrome.

We noticed she became very insistent about being covered up at all times. Even on holiday in hot countries she would wear a cardigan and leggings. She would no longer swim; something she used to love. She hated being in the sun so when we were abroad, if we could coax her to come out of the hotel room she would always sit in very shady areas. We did not realise at the time that she was suffering from heat intolerance and an inability to regulate her temperature.

Amy has enrolled in college twice. The first time it became too much for her and she was exhausted. The second time she fainted at the college and was too worried to go back in case it might happen again, especially on a staircase where she not only could injure herself but possibly others. We kept in touch with the college and were advised that she would be welcome to reapply after summer if her health improved; unfortunately, it deteriorated.

She lost her appetite completely in 2012 and still has to be reminded to eat something (she currently eats up to 2 very small 'meals' per day). This obviously has a knock-on effect with her energy levels. She visited a dietician who signed her off after 2 sessions as she was not concerned about Amy's weight. I still find it difficult to fathom that a dietician would focus purely on weight and not be concerned about the nutritional implications.

When I discovered the link between Amy's ongoing mystery illness and the HPV Vaccine, I researched and found the Facebook group, 'Parents of sons and daughters suffering illnesses after HPV vaccine,' which is administrated by Freda Birrell of the Association for HPV Vaccine Injured Daughters.

I found a wealth of support and further insights into possible side-effects, a number of which rang true with Amy. I noticed a number of her symptoms fit the symptoms of POTS. After printing out an NHS website definition of this to present to the GP, she agreed that Amy could possibly be presenting with this condition and arranged to have her referred to a cardiologist.

When we attended the pre-tilt-table consult, I regrettably mentioned our feeling that she may have POTS as a side effect of the vaccine, to which we got the usual roll of the eyes. When the time came for the actual tilt-table test, I was not allowed to be present. After the test was complete I was brought into the room to escort Amy out. She was perched on the bed completely disorientated. I asked if she could sit for a minute to come round but was told I would have to take her to the seats outside. I had to practically carry her out of the room with no assistance. Then we had to sit there for a good half-an-hour before she could even move. Amy was not diagnosed with POTS because she did not completely lose consciousness during the test. Amy later told me that she was so scared to pass out during the test that she did everything in her power to stop it from happening but was extremely close to it.

Amy has suffered from numbness in her limbs from quite early on after the vaccine. As of January 2016, Amy has been reliant on crutches indoors and a wheelchair on the odd occasions when she is fit enough to go out. Her walking had become so unsteady and she was too weak to keep herself upright unaided. Her legs would visibly shake and buckle under her.

One GP referred us to a physiotherapist. On the referral letter, she said that she had witnessed no problems with Amy's gait and that she just walked like an elderly person in fear of falling. She also stated myself and my mother were 'overly concerned'. During her session, the physiotherapist carried out a number of tests with Amy and said there was definitely a physical problem there. She sent a report of her findings to the GP, which resulted in Amy being referred to a neurologist.

Although the neurologist did not agree or disagree that the HPV Vaccine could be the cause, she came across as very sympathetic and quite interested in what we had to say, which felt great. She referred Amy for 2 MRI Scans to rule out MS but said she thought it was probably Functional Neurological Disorder.

When I went home, I researched FND, which I gather is really an umbrella term they are giving to people that are displaying autoimmune problems but they cannot find a physical problem with the brain. The research I found stated that a past psychological trauma is causing the sufferer to mentally block signals from the brain to the nerves. I also came across a script to diagnose FND – it was basically word for word everything the neurologist had said to us.

I found this very disheartening because it felt like she had already made her mind up that this is what Amy was suffering from and, therefore it had to be something traumatic that had happened in Amy's past that was causing her health issues rather than something physically attacking her body and brain.

Amy attended her MRI scans early December 2017. By April 2018, I had to chase up the results, which I was told were passed to our GP surgery back in January 2018. I had been told at the GP surgery the results would come to us directly. This did not happen. Finally in April 2018, I found out the results were negative for MS.

Amy was referred to a neurological physiotherapist. I was allowed to sit in on the first appointment, where I made it clear that we believed the HPV Vaccine was the root cause of all of Amy's health issues. The

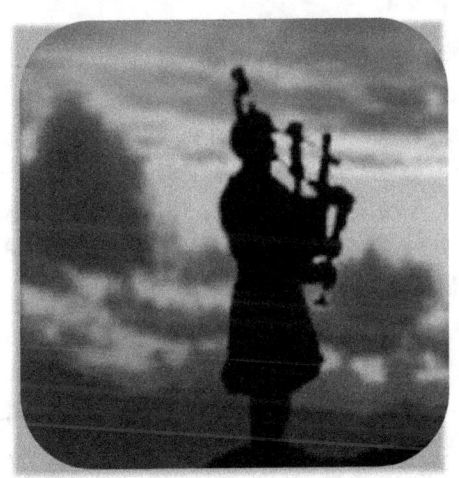

physiotherapist listened to our concerns but again would not comment on the cause. She said she would be unable to carry out any physiotherapy with Amy until we had the diagnosis or non-diagnosis of FND, however she was happy to work through some Cognitive Behavioural Therapy with Amy.

At the next appointment, although giving Amy the option on the spot, she made it quite clear I was not welcome in the following appointments. I reluctantly sat in the waiting area until the session finished an hour later. A couple of appointments later, Amy started to make some changes that would appear small to those who did not know her, but huge to us. Things like opening her room curtains or having something different if we treated ourselves to a takeaway.

Amy received her appointment for the FND consultant, to which I thought, "Great! One way or another her proper physiotherapy will start soon." However, when I collected Amy from her last physiotherapy appointment, she told me that she was not given an appointment and that the physiotherapist wanted to refer her to a psychiatrist or psychologist, but that Amy had to let her know if she wanted this.

Amy attended her appointment with the FND consultant, who has diagnosed her with FND. When we attended the appointment, the consultant asked what we thought the cause was. I mentioned the HPV Vaccine, she did not dismiss it, but again could not comment impartially.

She later said it would be best not to dwell on the cause as it would not help Amy. I stated I thought it was very important to know if the vaccine is able to cause FND. She then told me I should not vilify the vaccine, as she sees young women with Cervical Cancer, then turned to Amy saying, "At least you won't get that."

I was furious, not only was she giving my daughter a completely unfounded promise, she also seemed to be mocking the severity of what my daughter is going through, as well as our belief the vaccine was the root cause.

I responded that the vaccine has not been proven to prevent a single case of cancer, and is only supposed to protect against certain strains of HPV. I then told her we should leave the subject as we could end up debating at length, rather than focusing on Amy. The consultant said she would refer Amy back to physiotherapy, as well as a homeopath, though this could all take some time. We received an appointment to see the consultant again a year later.

I have been granted a career break from work and hope to help Amy to establish good eating patterns and routines so that she is able to become more independent. Hopefully, she will have some physiotherapy exercises in place so I can help her regain some strength and possibly overcome her mobility issues.

From the beginning of Amy's health deterioration, we have been in and out of doctor's surgeries countless times. In the beginning, before I knew that this vaccine was to blame, I would get so frustrated and almost always end up in tears when visiting the GPs, because it felt like it was a constant fight to try and find answers or help for Amy.

Once I made the connection, the appointments changed. I would mention the vaccine and be told 'it can't be that,' or 'it's just a teen thing'. This constant denial lead to me bringing the prescribing insert section 6.2, which outlined all the nasty side effects, to show one of the GPs, who blatantly ignored it.

I have gotten to the point where, if we see any new medical professional, I simply state "I know you are not allowed to agree with me, but after extensive research, we are of the opinion that Amy's health problems stem from the HPV vaccine, which she received just before she became ill."

I do not give them the chance to argue, but if they do, I am clued up enough now to state my case and to throw facts and figures at them. Maybe one day, we will see a medical professional who will actually listen to our concerns and admit the blatantly obvious truth.

Amy suffers from headaches almost constantly and has light sensitivity; she prefers to be in a dark room because of this. She has recently obtained transition lens glasses to see if this makes any difference for her.

Amy has no independence and rarely leaves the house, in fact the only time she really does is to attend doctor appointments.

The main side effects that Amy has been struggling with since she was given HPV vaccine are:

- Fainting Spells/Dizziness
- Irregular Heartbeat and Increased Heart Rate
- Shortness of Breath
- Complete Loss of Appetite
- Extreme Fatigue/Irregular Sleeping Patterns
- Depression – this has improved somewhat just from knowing why she is ill
- Severe Social Anxiety – this has improved over the past year
- Light & Noise Sensitivity
- Weakness
- Numbness of Lower Legs/Feet & 'Weird' feelings in arms
- Inability to Stand/Walk Unaided
- Constant Headaches
- General Feelings of Malaise
- Brain fog/cognitive impairment
- Inability to Regulate Temperature
- Functional Neurological Disorder

CHAPTER 3

Asia

Turkey

Turkey was the first Islamic country to implement a cervical cancer screening program using traditional pap smears in 2004. The national participation rate was only 1-2%. This was not nearly high enough to effectively control cervical cancer.[78] In 2013, HPV DNA testing was added to the conventional cytology program which was already in place. Current guidelines recommend screening by either pap smears or HPV DNA testing once every 5 years beginning at age 30. By 2017, more than 80% of the eligible population participated in the program, resulting in the National HPV Screening Laboratory processing between one and two million HPV DNA tests and 1.5 million cytology tests annually.

Between August 2014 and December 2015, more than 2 million HPV DNA tests were processed in the National HPV Screening Laboratory. High-risk HPV was only detected in 3.8% of the samples that had been analyzed. Even with such a low high-risk HPV prevalence rate, in the spring of 2017 the government was already debating on whether or not to add HPV vaccines to their cervical cancer prevention program.[79]

---

[78] Gultekin, Murat et al. "Initial results of population based cervical cancer screening program using HPV testing in one million Turkish women"; *International journal of cancer* vol. 142,9 (2017): 1952-1958; accessed March 2019

[79] Murat Gültekin, Baki Akgül; HPV screening in Islamic countries; Lancet

According to the ICO/IARC publication titled, *Turkey: Human Papillomavirus and Related Cancers, Fact Sheet 2018,* an estimated 2,356 new cervical cancer cases are diagnosed in Turkey each year.[80]

The same fact sheet states the cervical cancer rate in Turkey is 5.7/100,000. The latest official statistics that were available when the information sheet was prepared (2012) indicated the diagnosis rate varied greatly from one region to the next with a low of 3/100,000 and a high of 6.6/100,000. To bring this into perspective as far as 'health issues' are concerned, in 2012 the diagnosis rate for breast cancer was 53.8/100,000. Breast cancer was the number one cancer threat for the women of Turkey. Cervical cancer was much farther down the list at number 13.

For those unfamiliar with the ICO/IARC, the acronyms stand for Catalan Institute of Oncology (ICO) and the International Agency for Research on Cancer (IARC) respectively. According to the ICO page on PATH's Vaccine Resource Library, the information center was developed to 'accelerate the development and introduction of prophylactic HPV vaccines in countries with the highest burden of cervical cancer and reduce the incidence of this disease and related lesions among women.'[81]

The European Medicines Agency (EMA) approved Gardasil for use throughout the European Union, including Turkey, on 20 September 2006. Approval for Cervarix was granted one year later, on 20 September 2007. Both are currently approved for use in males and females age 9 and up to protect against cancer of the cervix or anus and precancerous lesions in the genital area (cervix, vulva, vagina or anus) which, according to the EMA, are caused by certain types of human papillomavirus (HPV). Gardasil is also said to protect against genital warts caused by specific types of human papillomavirus. [82, 83]

Gardasil 9 was approved for use on 9 June 2015 for use in males or females from age 9 for protection against lesions and cancers affecting

---

Correspondence Section; Volume 17; April 2017; accessed March 2019

[80] Turkey: Human Papillomavirus and Related Cancers, Fact Sheet 2018; ICO/IARC; accessed March 2019

[81] Vaccine Resource Library; PATH/ICO/IARC; accessed March 2019

[82] European Medicines Agency; Gardasil authorization details section; accessed March 2019

[83] European Medicines Agency; Cervarix authorization details section; accessed March 2019

the cervix, vulva, vagina and anus caused by vaccine-relevant HPV types as well as genital warts caused by specific HPV types.[84]

The government of Turkey does not have a formal HPV vaccination program. HPV vaccines are not currently included in the national immunization program. They are simply approved for use via private pay.

---

[84] European Medicines Agency; Gardasil 9 authorization details; accessed March 2019

Vaccine Injury or a Horror Movie?

By Su Asaad, Istanbul Turkey

"Lost years due to negligence of pharmaceutical companies"

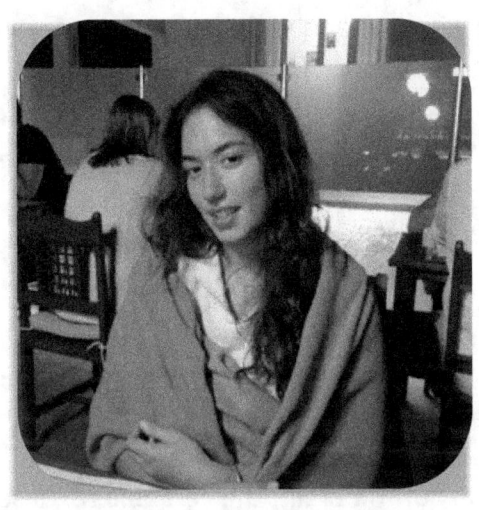

I am Su Asaad. I was born in Istanbul, Turkey in 1987. I've always been social and active. I began playing the piano at the age of 4. I would ride my bike, play basketball, taekwondo, do yoga, ballet, and dance, do hiking, and sing. I went to college in both Istanbul and Los Angeles and became a sound engineer. I had the privilege of working with world class musicians like Natalie Cole, The Cranberries, The Scorpions, Alan Parsons, and Burhan Ocala. I was also singing professionally... You may say, climbing up in my career. I always watched what I ate. I was never overweight. I've never had a serious health condition in my past.

That is until I got my three HPV vaccine injections. My aunt told my mom about this vaccine, and how it was said to prevent cancer and suggested my sister and I both should get it. When I consulted my doctor, she recommended the vaccine as well. It felt like a good idea to prevent cancer. So, we got the shots.

After my second shot, I remember saying 'something is wrong with my health'. After my third shot, I was almost going to faint. I got dizzy, but my doctor told me that it was normal, so I didn't worry about it. I was 23 years old. This was April 2011.

My sister was fine after the shots, but I began feeling constantly tired. I wanted to sleep all day, every day. I had just started a new job in May with probably the best Post Production Company in Turkey. I was hired to do sound design. It was my dream job!

But, during the very first week I felt out of breath nearly all of the time and was having heart palpitations very frequently. I had to tell the company that even though I really liked it there I was not physically ready to start a new job. They kindly told me to come back whenever I was ready.

Unfortunately, my symptoms worsened. I began having gastrointestinal issues like bloating, frequent urination, low blood pressure, neck pain and I had numbness in my fingers and feet, and sometimes in my face which really scared me.

By September, I began blacking out and with the other symptoms all together, I decided to go to a hospital. First to a gastroenterologist, who told me my problems were psychosomatic. Then a urologist, who told me to train myself by not going to the bathroom until there's an extreme urge. And finally, to a neurologist, because I thought there might be something wrong with my neck, causing these blackouts and numbness of my fingers.

After many examinations, the brain MRI report said "at the vertex level, on the left, distance of cerebrospinal fluid is increased" which they didn't consider to be important. The dorsal MRI's report said "2.7 mm at its largest, syringomyelia cavity between D1-D9". As a result, the doctor told me that I had Chiari malformation[85] (a serious neurological disorder where the bottom part of the brain, the cerebellum, descends out of the skull and crowds the spinal cord, putting pressure on both the brain and spine and causing many symptoms) and syringomyelia[86] (spinal cord cyst) and recommended a surgery for me. A spinal surgery sounded very scary.

I showed my MRI's to other doctors, they told me I was fine, and this would not cause me any trouble. I stopped going to doctors for a while.

I was feeling fatigued all the time, my fiancé and I would go out somewhere, but when we arrived, I would beg him to let me stay in the car and sleep. We began dating after the second shot when I didn't have nearly this much fatigue. So, he couldn't understand what was going on either.

I began paying extra attention to my diet, I would consume less carbs, I would exercise, but by summer 2012 my eyelids began twitching in addition to all of the other new symptoms.

---

[85] https://www.conquerchiari.org/index.html
[86] https://csfinfo.org/education/physician-information/syringomyelia/

On August 2012 I had my first seizure. I didn't know it was a seizure until later. We had had a perfect day. We were at my aunt's ranch and I was preparing the table for supper. Suddenly I had a really strong 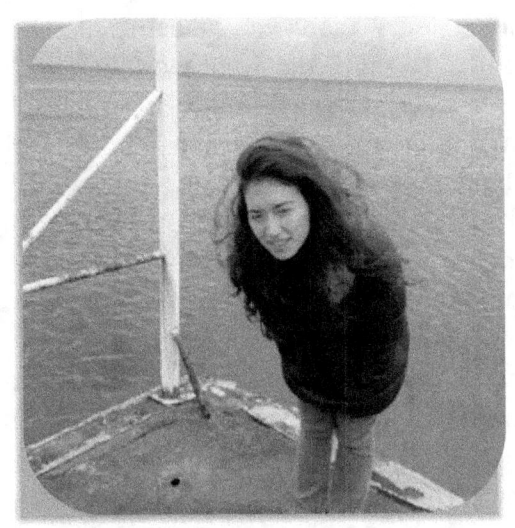 sensation of Déjà vu, which wouldn't go away when I looked away. Everywhere I looked I would have the feeling 'I lived this exact moment before' and also a feeling that 'something bad will happen really soon'. An energy from my gut to my head raced up and my brain was on fire. I called my aunt and my fiancé, crying, trying to tell them what was happening. The whole episode lasted maybe a minute but, I was very scared. It couldn't be an anxiety attack, I was very happy just a moment before.

During the week, this happened 6 more times, before I saw a neurologist. The Déjà vu sensation, the warm energy from my gut to head, as if I was going to throw up but I would never throw up, then my brain would, I would best describe the feeling as 'fry'. Sometimes, during the attack I would feel like I would not be able to swallow anything, as if the back of my tongue was swelling. And usually, but not always, within an hour of the minute-long seizures a headache would reach its peak and ache for at least an hour. I've never had headaches in my life. I've never had a need to use a pain killer until that time.

The neurologist I went to didn't ask for an MRI, since I already had one from last year. I showed her my old MRI's and told her about the syringomyelia diagnosis. She said that has nothing to do with this. She had me take an EEG test and told me the EEG report showed nothing significant. For the record, the EEG report states, "Cerebral bioelectric activity normal, mild functional disorder on left anterior temporal area evoked by hyperventilation."

By that time, I had begun to do my own research. I knew this experience was called 'temporal lobe epilepsy'.

My family was very irritated when they heard the word epilepsy. My mom kept shutting me up, saying I was fine. This made me feel even worse, because once they accepted the situation, I knew they would help me find a solution. Denial would not get me anywhere near a cure.

The doctor prescribed an epilepsy medicine called Lamictal. She made me use it for three months. Not only did it not work, my seizures increased up to three times a day. I was feeling like I was a fully charged battery and within one minute the charge would deplete leaving me feeling exhausted and mentally devastated.

Imagine this happening three times a day. I was frustrated. After three months, I called my doctor again to say that the meds were not working. I was very disappointed to hear her say, "Then, go to a psychologist."

I did go to a psychologist, and many other specialists, even to people who called themselves healers. There was no improvement whatsoever.

When I was having the seizures, my family would tell me to stop panicking and that there was nothing to be afraid of. This drove me crazy because my seizures had nothing to do with panic. They would happen when I was happy or sad regardless of my mood. Seizures would even wake me up from a sound sleep. While sleeping, all of a sudden a racing heart and a burning sensation from my gut to brain would wake me up and afterwards I would feel beat up.

I would pray to God, cry to God, nothing was helping me. Sometimes, I would wake up feeling as if something from the inside was pinching my throat, like someone was strangling me.

My life had become a horror movie and no one could understand me. I think that was the worst part, being alone... Even though there were people around me, no one really understood. Everyone thought all my new medical symptoms were psychosomatic.

November 2012, my first biofeedback session.

Ever since my childhood, I had been interested in frequency therapies. My mom had a friend who referred her to a bio resonance session, which I also got to experience. It was so much fun. I got to learn a lot about my body. By the time I became a sound engineer, I had learned much about healing frequencies and brain waves. I had researched many kinds of machines but never the quantum biofeedback system.

A week after my first biofeedback session, I realized I had not suffered a seizure for one whole week. I had not expected this all. They had not told me I could heal, or give me any hope that this was even a possibility. After this shocking development, I decided to stop going to the psychologist, and continue biofeedback sessions instead.

For the first three sessions, I went every week. Then I began going every two weeks, and finally decreased sessions to once a month. I was feeling lively again!

I was finally able to begin working as a production coordinator and accomplished a lot of good work.

In 2013, I decided to become a biofeedback therapist and went to Victor Babes University in Timisoara, Romania. There, I've learned neuro-electrophysiology, neuroanatomy and biofeedback. I became my own therapist. I was seizure free for another year.

In December 2014, I was food poisoned and the seizures came back. I thought the inflammation probably triggered the return of my symptoms.

During the next couple of weeks, I saw another neurologist. This time my diagnosis was 'Migraine, with an aura'. Apparently it was irrelevant that I didn't always have headaches after seizures. This neurologist's treatment was to keep an 'attack diary' which I did. Within a couple weeks, I was again able to stop my seizures using biofeedback.

I was working as a biofeedback specialist now, and the therapies were very successful. People with anxiety or depression would heal within a session or two. Even people with autoimmune disease such as Multiple Sclerosis, Hashimoto's or psoriasis would start healing after the first session. My machine was doing a great job controlling inflammation, so was I, controlling the machine. Allergies would heal, even the extreme ones. I was able to find the causes of my patients' diseases. Sometimes that cause would be trauma, sometimes a pathogen, and sometimes an environmental toxicity. No matter what the cause, improvements were made.

Unfortunately, I had a seizure again on January 2016. At the time I had begun eating too many sweets which probably caused inflammation.

Upon a friend's recommendation, I went to see a new neurologist. She wanted an MRI with an Epilepsy Protocol, which came out fine. As the MRI report said, "No evidence of mesial temporal sclerosis was detected." But, the EEG report stated, "Mild neuronal hyper excitability in the left frontal-temporal region on the basis of bioelectric disorganization."

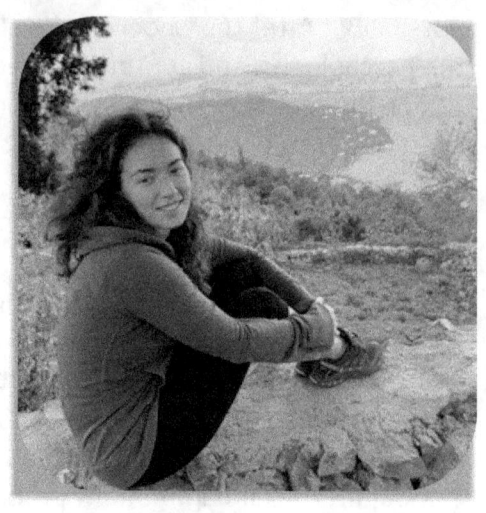

My neurologist told me she went down to talk to the MRI technician herself to make sure there was no physiological finding and was then convinced there was not. She then told me that there might be something on a cellular level, which would be very painful to detect, so we passed that option.

At my request we tested for some viruses. All IgM's were within acceptable limits. She told me normally she would prescribe a medicine in a situation like this, but, somehow I was managing the symptoms. "So, keep doing what you're doing to prevent the seizures," she said. And I did. She began sending people who don't respond to medicines to my biofeedback sessions.

Keep doing what I am doing is of course not just biofeedback. I have learned the KETOGENIC diet and intermittent fasting is also helpful.

Doctor David Perlmutter perfectly explains that 'neurogenesis' is what we want. One needs to consume lots of water (natural spring or mineral), magnesium (citrate), sodium (Himalayan salt), potassium (avocado), and lots of healthy fats like coconut oil, virgin olive oil and grass-fed butter on this diet.

I am also exercising, doing fitness training, and a lot of hiking. Hiking is the best. Exercise is really good for controlling inflammation.

In August 2016 I got married. It was the happiest day of my life. I took a break from my diet and was fine. I was eating normal foods, consuming some sugar from time to time.

Then in October 2016, I had an abnormal pap smear. The biopsy results came out to be CIN3 "High grade dysplasia / In situ squamous cell carcinomas."

My doctor told me there is no recovering from this and that my only option is surgery. "Please see a gynecologic oncologist and have the LEEP procedure," she said.

I panicked and immediately scheduled an appointment to see a gynecologic oncologist. The doctor was very unconvincing. This HPV was a DNA virus, and if we do this procedure, it was very likely the cancer could reoccur later on. So, this was a symptomatic solution.

Instead of cutting my cervix out, I needed it to heal first, and then 'keep it up' to prevent the disease from returning. I needed to starve the pathogens by cutting out their 'food' supply, which is sugar/grains/legumes/fructose. And I needed to boost my immune system, instead of cutting out a piece of me.

So, I refused the procedure, telling my doctor I took full responsibility. I supplemented with L-lysine 2000mg a day for 3 months. Beta-Glucan became my best friend. I worked with the biofeedback machine for degeneration, and viruses. Exercised. As a result, I healed my cervix completely. My doctor was shocked, she wasn't expecting this at all.

After the dysplasia, the puzzle pieces began to fit in place. All this time, I kept going back in my mind, trying to find the beginning of my health's deterioration and finally found the answer. HPV vaccinated people have higher rates of developing high-grade dysplasia. I also found out that many girls after HPV vaccination were suffering severe neurological diseases. Healthy, active and lively girls. As I read, I was more and more convinced the HPV vaccine played a big part, either causing or triggering my new medical symptoms.

Nevertheless, I believe I am one of the lucky ones. I know the neurological repair I experienced after using the biofeedback machine helped me recover.

Maybe some of the new medical symptoms I experienced were because of the high aluminium content in the vaccine. Maybe the heavy-metal detox from using the biofeedback machine saved me.

The biggest question remaining is, why was I injured and my sister wasn't?

I believe there are a few possibilities. One, in 2009 I got shingles which went away in a week after being prescribed Zovirax. That probably made my nerves more sensitive. Two, I am susceptible to cold sores and she is not. And three, I had warts on my feet when I was a kid -three or four small ones- and they didn't go away until 2008. In 2008, I began consuming L-lysine regularly to prevent cold sores and surprisingly within a month or two, I noticed all my warts were gone. So, my nerves were more susceptible to pathogens and toxins than my sister was.

I have spent thousands and thousands of dollars on examinations and therapies. I have fallen behind on my career. My family and my husband struggled. There is nothing that can make up for the time I have lost.

I want this vaccine to be taken off the market. I don't want any more young people to get hurt. I want justice and I want compensation for me and all of the other injured girls and boys.

Japan

Cervarix was licensed in Japan in 2009. Gardasil was licensed in 2011. Both vaccines were partially funded by various regional governments until October 2010 when central and local governments launched a temporary funding program.[87]

Despite the subsidies, HPV vaccines did not come into widespread use until after revisions to Japan's Preventive Vaccination Law took effect in April 2013. This change put HPV vaccines on the national schedule with a recommendation for use in 12 to 16-year-old girls.

Less than two months later, on the 14th of June 2013, Japan's Ministry of Health, Labor, and Welfare rescinded this recommendation when more than half of the 3.28 million citizens injected with Gardasil or Cervarix reported adverse reactions.[88] The government announced both vaccines would remain available for use and subsidized by the government. However, they should no longer be proactively recommended nor promoted. Ironically, this occurred one day after the World Health Organization (WHO) declared the HPV vaccine safe.[89]

According to the Center for Strategic and International Studies (CSIS), "The MHLW's suspension of active recommendation of HPV vaccination in Japan has negatively impacted public trust in the vaccine."[90] This statement was published in 2015, apparently in an attempt to shame Japan into altering their position on HPV vaccinations.

---

[87] Press Release; Merck receives approval to market Gardasil, Zolina and Cubicin; European Pharmaceutical Review; 1 July 2011; accessed March 2019

[88] Staff writer; Analysis: Experts at loss over pain from cervical cancer vaccination; The Asahi Shimbun; 2013; excerpt available on SaneVax.org

[89] Wilson, Rose; Paterson, Pauline; Larson, Heidi J.; Vaccination in Japan-Issues and Options; CSIS Global Health Policy Center; May 2014; accessed March 2019

[90] Larson, Heidi, et al; HPV Vaccination in Japan: The Continuing Debate and Global Impacts; CSIS Global Health Policy Center; April 2015; accessed March 2019

Two years later in December of 2017, the Global Advisory Committee on Vaccine Safety issued a similar condemnation stating, "The circumstances in Japan, where the occurrence of chronic pain and other symptoms in some vaccine recipients has led to suspension of the proactive recommendation for routine use of vaccine in the national immunization program, warrants additional comment. Review of clinical data by the national expert committee led to a conclusion that symptoms were not related to the vaccine, but it has not been possible to reach consensus to resume HPV vaccination. As a result, young women are being left vulnerable to HPV-related cancers that otherwise could be prevented. As GACVS has noted previously, policy decisions based on weak evidence, leading to lack of use of safe and effective vaccines, can result in real harm."[91]

Logically speaking, this seems like a rather odd statement particularly when you consider the fact that the latest WHO sponsored HPV Fact Sheet for Japan states that only 'about 1.9%' of the women in Japan are estimated to harbor HPV 16/18 infections at any given time, and 'only 52.9% of invasive cervical cancers are attributed to HPVs 16/18.'[92]

In spite of the worldwide pressure being exerted to compel Japanese officials to change their mind, the government recommendation for HPV vaccine use has not been reinstated.

Perhaps it has something to do with the fact that under Japanese law bureaucrats found to have neglected their duty to inform medical consumers of serious risks involved with taking medicines, vaccines and other medical products can be prosecuted and severely punished.[93]

---

[91] GACVS-Statement on Safety of HPV vaccines; 17 Dec 2017; accessed March 2019

[92] Japan: Human Papillomavirus and Related Cancers, Fact Sheet 2018; ICO/IARC/WHO; accessed March 2019

[93] Erickson, N; HPV Vaccines: Japan requires disclosure of side effects; SaneVax Inc.; 29 Aug 2013; accessed March 2019

HPV Vaccine: Cervarix Injury

By Mika Matsufuji, Mother of injured child and Representative of the Japanese Association of Cervical Cancer Vaccine Injured People (since March 25, 2013)

My daughter, Mai (not her real name) was in her first year of Junior High School when she was administered the HPV vaccine, Cervarix. She was only 12 years old. We had no idea how drastically our lives would change that year.

Before Vaccination:

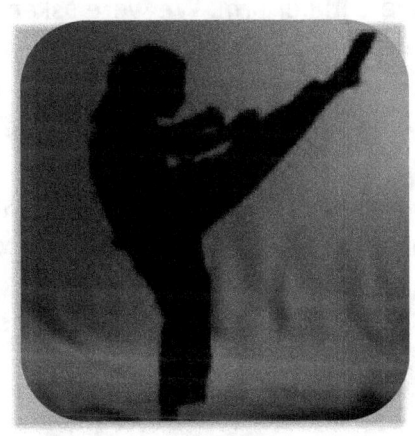

Mai was attending a local state junior high school with the traditional curriculum with the addition of art club as an extracurricular activity. During a school sports day event in June of 2011, she came in first in the 100 meter run. She was a quiet girl who enjoyed reading books.

In addition to normal school activities, Mai began to learn Karate and traditional Japanese dance while still in the first grade of elementary school. In the third grade, she added piano lessons to her after school activities.

My daughter was generally very healthy. She was hospitalized when she was in the fifth grade because of abdominal pain. She tested positive for E. coli and stayed in the hospital for approximately two weeks. Several months after that, she developed appendicitis and was admitted to the hospital again. The doctor said that the abdominal pain she experienced before the previous hospital visit might have also been due to problems with her appendix. Other than these two incidents, she had no history of hospitalization.

Immediately After HPV Vaccination:

Mai received her first injection of the HPV vaccine, Cervarix, on September 16, 2011. This was followed by the administration of a vaccine for Japanese Encephalitis on September 29, 2011. She had no obvious problems after either of these shots.

Then, came the injection we will never forget. It was October 19, 2011 and the weather was beautiful. Around 4 o'clock in the afternoon, Mai and I visited a local pediatric clinic where she received her second dose of Cervarix. There was no remarkable event when the needle was inserted.

The doctor asked her, "Are you OK?"

She replied, "I am fine."

Immediately after the vaccine was administered and the needle was removed, she started to feel a numbness in her arm. We were asked to wait in the waiting room, but before Mai could get to a chair, she complained to the nurse of a strange feeling in her body. We were sent back to the examination room. However, we were just told to keep watching to see how it would go, then sent home.

The numbness continued for the whole day. During the night, she got a headache and fever. Her whole left arm (the one the shot was given in) started to get red and swell while the pain increased.

The clinic telephoned that night to ask how she was. I told them about the numbness, swelling, etc.… and said I would continue to watch her.

Adverse Reactions Thereafter:

The next day, she had a severe back ache. I noticed that her shoulder and the left side of her back appeared to be raised. The swelling and redness in her left arm increased and she was experiencing a burning sensation along with severe pain.

In the morning, I telephoned the doctor who had administered the vaccine and we went to the clinic. Without examining Mai well, the doctor said, "We cannot treat her here anymore. We have just made an appointment for your daughter at a general hospital nearby."

We immediately went to the general hospital and saw a doctor. The pediatrician who saw Mai could not give a diagnosis. Later, we would see a neurologist.

The swelling in her arm and body pain were so severe Mai was hospitalized in a pediatric ward.

She was hospitalized for ten days, but there was no improvement. She was referred to another university hospital for treatment of the pain.

On the day Mai was discharged from the hospital, we went to the anesthesiology department of the second university hospital. The doctor there did now know about the vaccine and prescribed pregabalin capsules and clonazepam. He also ordered an MRI, X-rays and standard blood tests. A diagnosis of CRPS was given.

As we were heading home in the early evening, the pain started to spread to her legs. Walking became difficult. By night-time, she could not walk at all. When we informed the hospital about her inability to walk, the doctor said that it could not be CRPS and could not be handled in the anesthesiology department of the outpatient pain clinic. We were told to go back to the original hospital and that the doctor at this clinic could not see her anymore.

After this, Mai could not go upstairs to a bedroom. We make her bed in a room downstairs by laying a mattress on the floor. Mai became bedridden apart from hospital visits.

When she needed to go to a toilet, I dragged the mattress with Mai on top of it, supported her and lifted her body to allow her to sit on the seat. I carried meals to her bed and helped her eat. She could not even sit up to eat.

Changes in Conditions:

The pain in her vaccinated left arm started to become permanent and other parts of her body started to ache randomly. The pain in her legs intensified and the numbness spread.

Around six weeks after vaccination, she began to experience memory impairment along with acalculia (loss of the ability to perform simple math calculations). At one point, her memory impairment was so severe that she could not remember names of her family members, sometimes even her own. She began to experience involuntary movements in her legs and at times foam would discharge from her mouth when she was sleeping.

Gradually, she found it difficult to sleep and showed a movement like an REM sleep disorder when she was sleeping. Around this time, the swelling in her left arm started to subside. The pain in her legs also began to alleviate a little. However, she now began to experience a severe sleep disorder. As soon as she began to fall asleep, her arms and legs would begin to move involuntarily, kicking and punching. She also started sleep walking. These sleep disorders would repeat nightly and continue into the early morning hours. Eventually, she would be able to go to sleep then wake up after lunch time.

Her symptoms were so severe she was again hospitalized for more tests, including an electroencephalogram, cerebrospinal fluid tests, etc. This time she was in the hospital for ten days. The tests revealed that when the unusual sleep behavior disorder was occurring, her brain was awake. The REM sleep disorder was ruled out and the conclusion was a 'disease of unknown cause'. During this stay in the hospital, her involuntary movements were so severe that the restraining straps holding her to a bed were torn in only a week.

This condition continued every day for three to four months.

Around this time, in addition to the pains, she developed a multitude of new symptoms including loss of consciousness, allodynia (pain from stimuli that would not normally produce pain), sleep disorder, panic attacks which caused her to cry and become violent, back pain, skin rashes on her palms, soles of her feet and head, numbness throughout her body, memory impairment, dysphagia (difficulty swallowing), decreased level of platelets. These abnormal conditions continued.

She started to feel that the light was too glaring and needed to wear ski goggles all of the time. Even so, she still felt the light was too strong. We had to darken her room by using light-shielding curtains. This problem continued for about three years.

After episodes of losing consciousness, her vision became green and she was frightened by hallucinations. She needed someone with her at all times.

Furthermore, there was a period of two to three weeks when she developed severe allergies to all food. We had to rush her to the emergency room almost every day.

2013, Two Years after Vaccination:

Mai still suffered from severe headaches. She would lose consciousness multiple times per day. She had almost constant pain throughout her body, taste disorders, severe light sensitivity, allodynia below her knees to the point where she could not dip her legs in a bath, dysphagia, double vision, tinnitus (ringing in her ears), walking disability severe enough to require the use of a wheelchair, acalculia, memory impairment, chronic fatigue, sleep disorders, pain in the left side of her back, left upper back remained raised, and CRPS.

Therapies received to date:

- Steroid pulse
- Chinese herbal medicine
- Prescription medicines for pain, such as pregabalin capsules and clonazepam
- Chiropractic treatments (need to be cautious since licensing is not required in Japan)
- Tapping
- B spot therapy (a method for treating inflammation of nasopharynx behind nose and throat with 0.5% zinc chloride using a long cotton swab)
- Aeration (a treatment to improve the passage of air through ears)
- High-dose IV Vitamin C
- Dietary intervention for allergies
- Prescribed medicine such as Vitamin B's for supplementing vitamin deficiencies
- Immuno-adsorption plasmapheresis

2017: Five-and-a-half Years after Vaccination

Mai still suffers from sleep disorders, skin rashes that cover her whole body, double vision (although somewhat less severe), involuntary movements (decreased to once every other week), severe headaches, swelling and pain in palms and soles, raised left shoulder and back, loss of consciousness (reduced to about every five days), back pain, heaviness and tiredness, POTS, chemical sensitivities, electromagnetic wave sensitivity, food allergies, menstruation disturbance, dyskinesia-like symptoms in both feet, restless leg syndrome, tinnitus, panic attacks (although somewhat better than before), can walk sometimes, but still needs a wheelchair.

Mai has been hospitalized eleven times since her second injection of Cervarix.

The hospitals we visited when her new medical conditions first appeared admitted the vaccine injury because she started to have new health problems immediately after the second injection.

However, hospitals we visited for treatments later often treated us disgracefully. We actually had doctors say:

- "You did not want to go to school, did you? It is a psychogenic disease characteristic to adolescents. I will refer you to a good psychiatric department."
- "Because Mai is being seen in a university hospital, I do not want to see her."
- "I cannot figure this out either. Hmmm, I wonder what it is."
- "I cannot see her with such mysterious symptoms. Why have you come here?"

School:

Our family's first priority has been trying to improve Mai's health. She could hardly go to school for a year-and-three-months after the adverse reactions began. After that, she started to go to school as often as her medical conditions would allow. When the new medical symptoms became worse, she could not attend school at all.

Her memory impairment, acalculia, panic attacks, involuntary movements, episodes of loss of consciousness, etc. made it extremely difficult for her to attend school on any sort of regular basis.

We hoped there was some kind of support from the government, but even if there had been, school would be very difficult for my daughter.

On the rare occasions when she could go to school, she would experience involuntary movements, severe headaches, or loss of consciousness. I often received telephone calls asking me to pick her up. She could not go on sleepovers, one-day trips, graduation, etc.

When she was old enough to attend senior high school, her only option was correspondence school. The traditional school personnel were very considerate and understanding. Mai was able to graduate from high school.

She is hoping to go to a university, but it will be difficult for her to attend lessons every day. We are thinking about the option of a correspondence university. As things are this year, she could not even go to an examination hall for her university entrance exams. She is working to prepare for the possibility of taking the entrance exam next year.

Local Government: Suginami Ward, Tokyo

We received two visits from local government officials after the adverse reactions began. There was also a visit to the hospital where Mai was staying, but in a ward assembly the head of the health care center department, who had personally visited us, replied to a question about adverse reactions to HPV vaccines stating, "There is no case of severe adverse reactions within this ward."

This statement became a problem later when a case of severe adverse reactions in Suginami ward became public via a news broadcast. A doctor working in the hospital where Mai was staying issued a written diagnosis stating that her new medical conditions were a reaction to Cervarix.

The head of health care center department admitted a lie in a subsequent ward assembly and corrected his previous words.

The Future?

We want to know whether Mai's new medical conditions will ever be completely cured. It is heart-breaking to see her not being able to fully enjoy her teenage years the same way other children do. It is difficult to watch her try and cope with memory impairment. Sometimes memories that seemed to have been lost come back, sometimes they do not. It is hard for parents to understand how this can happen.

She spent years taking piano lessons, but now cannot read music scores or understand musical notes. This ability has not returned at all.

We want to know whether her pain will be cured in the future. She still experiences losses of consciousness once every five or ten days. It is almost like epilepsy. She suddenly freezes and falls to the floor like a rag-doll without any warning symptoms. During these attacks, her eyeballs are shaking back and forth. Her doctors say it is not epilepsy. She cannot bathe without assistance because these episodes are so dangerous. When her health is poor, these episodes happen several times per hour. She requires the attendance of other people all the time.

She still has the constant tiredness, feeling of exhaustion and heaviness. She always suffers from a backache. Normal life is not possible for Mai.

Our only hope is the early establishment of a successful treatment protocol. We want our daughter to have her life back.

Sharne's Cervarix Injury

By her Mother, Machiko Kurosaki

Sharne was born in 1998. Her childhood health issues included: pervasive developmental disorder (PDD), a form of Asperger's, infantile asthma, atopic dermatitis, pyelitis (inflammation of the renal pelvis), otitis media, Candida, hemolytic streptococcus, pneumonia, warts, FMF (periodic fever syndrome), agrochemical sensitivity and repeated stomatitis. Despite these issues as an infant and child, she was thriving and doing well. After the administration of Cervarix, this all changed.

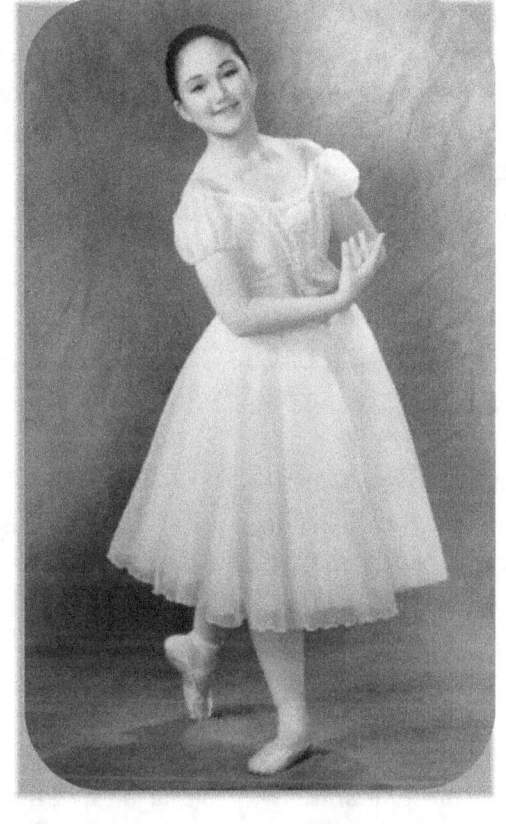

I wrote my daughter's story originally under the title, "Walking on the Edge of a Sword: Cervarix Injury in Japan."

The details of her physical and mental condition up to June 2014 are covered in this article and can be viewed at https://www.hormonesmatter.com/walking-edge-sword-cervarix-injury-japan/.

The following information is an update to that article. I write this hoping our experience searching for successful treatment protocols will help other parents who are in a similar situation. I want to let other parents know there is hope.

My daughter Sharne was 12-years-old when she had her first Cervarix injection on the 27th of July 2011. Later that day her eyes became red, three days later a rash appeared on her face and body, six days later she had folliculitis above ears, and fifteen days later she complained of headache when standing up. Her asthma attacks came back for the first time in seven years. But, I did not connect these symptoms to Cervarix, and took her to a doctor for the second injection. Due to her asthma flaring up, the injection was postponed. Around this time, Sharne also had nose bleeds, diarrhea, skin infections, temporomandibular arthrosis, parotitis, etc.... Stomatitis and diarrhea with abdominal pain were a problem every day.

Sharne was a quiet, independent, and determined girl who always looked after herself. She enjoyed reading, studying and running. In spite of the new health problems, she kept going as usual. Nobody around her noticed any change and did not connect these symptoms with Cervarix.

Sharne had her second Cervarix injection on the 17th of October 2011, and then her third Cervarix injection on 26th March 2012. Soon after the third injection, she developed muscle weakness, hyperpnoea and malaise and her comprehension level deteriorated. Sharne still kept going as normal until one day in mid-July she said to me, "I want to go to see a doctor."

Her pediatrician said, "There is definitely something wrong with her," and Sharne was referred to a doctor with knowledge of immunology.

From this point on, Sharne received many treatments including oral steroids (October to December 2012), IVIG (September 2013), steroid pulse therapy (February and March 2014), and immune-adsorption plasmapheresis (IAPP) (May 2014).

In the hospital where Sharne had a steroid pulse therapy in February and March 2014, she also had blood and CSF tests. The values of a lot of cytokines in the results were very high and the doctor told us that Sharne should see an immunologist.

In May 2014, the test results revealed that she was positive for anti-ganglioside antibodies, so Sharne went to a hospital in order to receive an immune-adsorption therapy (IAPP) for the first time. IAPP is a therapy which removes pathogens, cytokines, complements, and autoantibodies that are uncontrollably high in the blood.

Her depression, involuntary movement, irritability, malaise, etc. were very serious around this time. After the IAPP, the involuntary movement decreased although spasms and tremors started. Her motivation came back and she returned to her gentle and cheerful self. Sharne could even run for a short distance and ride a bicycle during the first week after the IAPP.

The IgE value in her blood test was 498 IU/ml, which had been greater than 1600 IU/ml before. Most surprisingly, the erythrocyte sedimentation rate, which shows chronic inflammation, decreased to 2 mm/h after IAPP. It had been around 30 mm/h after receiving Cervarix. 50% hemolytic complement activity (CH-50) was 48.1, which had been greater than 60. The IgD value also decreased and the slight degree of chronic fever started to go down.

Although the test results showed improvement, malaise and hypersomnia returned one week after the treatment, and Sharne was sleeping longer and longer and still being tired upon awakening. The erythrocyte sedimentation rate then started to increase. When I showed her cytokine test results to an immunologist around this time, he suggested we test for anti-NMDA receptor antibodies and the result was positive.

My husband and I tried everything available. Around this time, Sharne received a high dose IV vitamin C (distilled water 150ml, B1:120mg, B2:2mg, B3:40mg, B5:250mg, B6: 120mg, C: 12.5g, 0.5M magnesium sulfate: 5ml). Many girls in Japan had good results from this therapy, but each time Sharne received the treatment, her back and hip pain worsened, the gastrointestinal pain increased, she lost appetite, and she looked more tired.

We also heard about the importance of diet, Sharne has taken silica water and probiotics. I was brought up in a traditional farmer's community and was always careful of what we ate even before Sharne had Cervarix. I never used chemical seasoning. Sharne never had coffee, Coca Cola, or other sweetened beverages. Confectionery with chemicals and sweeteners were not included in her normal diet. Her grandparents grow rice and vegetables organically.

In August 2014, Sharne developed severe malaise and was hospitalized again for her second IAPP. At the time of the previous hospitalization, she was using a wheelchair due to systemic pain, which began after the steroid pulse therapy. This time, although she had malaise, hypersomnia and weakness in her left body, she chose to walk into the hospital dragging her leg.

Since the effect of previous IAPP treatment did not last long, I wanted Sharne to take an immunosuppressant this time. Her doctor did not agree because Sharne did not appear to be seriously bad despite very poor test results. Her doctor was not willing to give any drug that had a potential risk involved. I thought her inflammation had been suppressed by the steroid and IVIG she received earlier that year when she had a brain inflammation-like state, and this was the reason that her physical state looked better than it would be expected from her test results. When tested in August, anti-ganglioside antibodies were negative, and in December anti-NMDA receptor antibodies were also negative. The immunologist said that these antibodies might increase again when the vaccine antibodies increased, so Sharne should have blood tests regularly.

Unfortunately, after this IAPP treatment a lot of symptoms such as slight fever, stomatitis, blurred vision, restless legs, hyperventilation, headache, chest pain, back and hip pain, ear ringing, and memory problems were appearing at the same time. An encephalopathy-like state that had happened two years ago began again. Sharne's thoughts became very cloudy, she could not get up at all, and her speech deteriorated. Her awareness was still unclear the following morning. Around lunch time, she tried to get up but could not even keep sitting up without support. Her awareness seemed to come back a little, but she could not speak at all. That night clonic convulsion started during non-REM sleep. This occurred every night thereafter. The level and duration gradually worsened.

We tried a neurological medication, but it was effective only for a short time. The symptoms returned soon, so we stopped the medication. An EEG was done while Sharne was having involuntary movements, but there was no sign of epileptic seizure activity. The involuntary movement intensified night after night. Each time she lost consciousness after the involuntary movement, her memory got worse. I was very worried. I heard that many other girls who were suffering from the side effects of this vaccine in Japan had lost memories and the memories did not come back.

This terrible thing happened to my daughter as well. One day, she thought I was an elephant and kicked me. When she came to herself, she could not remember what had happened. She seemed to have lost her long-term memory and could not remember names of her family including her own name, address, birthday, and telephone number. Children with epilepsy do not lose memories even after they are left to sleep subsequent to seizures. However, children injured with this vaccine are losing their memories.

I tried to wake her up as quickly as possible after she lost consciousness. I tried to imprint her with memories. Even during middle of the night, I tried to imprint her with names of her family, relationships, her birthday, her grandparents' names and important people I do not want her to forget. I repeated everything until she could remember them.

One morning, she could not remember things I taught during the night. I felt I was going to go mad with despair. There are many parents in Japan who still share this exact feeling.

When Sharne started losing memories, she was concerned about it. She wrote down names of her family and friends and relationships on the back of hospital meal tickets and taped them to her bed rails. She gradually stopped doing this, and she started to confuse her own name with her friend's name.

Finally, when I corrected her, she argued saying, "Mother is making a mistake with my name."

Soon after, rigor and muscle weakness started, and she lost the ability to use chopsticks. Her involuntary movements started to occur even during the day. It affected her lower legs the most. She could not support her own head, so I supported her head and pushed her wheelchair.

One doctor said carelessly to her, "Your legs were standing on the bed, I cannot understand why you cannot stand up and walk? It is not muscle weakness."

By this time, she could not remember the date or who she met. She kept complaining of blurred and double vision.

I was really concerned Sharne was suffering from brain damage. I wanted her to remember her family. I lived every day as if I were lying down on a bed of nails. I worried more about brain damage than trunk dysfunction or articulation disorder. I thought I was going mad.

As one last recourse, I asked her doctor to please remember the affection his parents had given to him when they brought him up.

Her doctor proposed steroid pulse therapy to stop the existing inflammation. However, Sharne refused to have it because the steroid pulse therapy she received in February and March was not only ineffective but also caused systemic pain. I needed to convince her. Sharne had been on a gluten-free diet after reading about weak blood brain barrier. I traded the steroid pulse treatment with her for her favorite pork bun, which was made from wheat, and she agreed to receive steroid pulse.

It appeared to work. Although there were still involuntary movements, rigor and muscle weakness in lower legs, I felt the inflammation had been stopped by the steroid pulse.

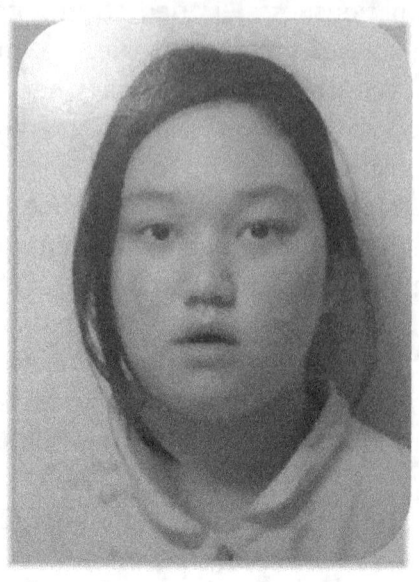

At this time, a doctor who read my blog e-mailed me with concern and told me that if Sharne were his daughter, he would give her vitamin C. I opened a vitamin C supplement, mixed it with a juice, and let Sharne drink it. That night, her loss of consciousness, which had been occurring every night, stopped.

While in the hospital, Sharne was receiving rehabilitation therapy. Once she learned how to move between a bed and a wheelchair, she did everything she could to lighten the burden on me. She was trying hard to recover, but when she overheard somebody saying that she was pretending not to be able to walk, she was hurt and started to ask me to take her home.

One time, after it became dark, with desolation she tried to climb a fence and escape. She spent several hours wandering around in the dark. We decided to go home. Doctors were worried about her going home with her present conditions. However, since I was a qualified caregiver, I knew how to treat a patient, and thought we could manage with the help of our care service.

After returning home, Sharne kept suffering from involuntary movements, muscle weakness, and rigor, but about two months later her lower legs started to show some strength. Around this time, Dr. Derrick Lonsdale kindly responded to my article on Hormonesmatter and suggested Sharne might have mitochondria dysfunction and might benefit from taking L-arginine. I had printed out his comment and showed it to Sharne's doctor. Her doctor said that we have nothing we can do at the moment and we would try everything that seems good with low risk and prescribed L-arginine together with biotin and levocarnitine.

Although these two were unknown to me at that time, I discovered later they are nutrients that regulate intestinal mucous membrane and protect and grow neurons. Sharne found they had positive effects on her and still takes those supplements occasionally for improvement of muscle weakness. She also takes vitamin C almost every day, and a pomegranate component as I heard that it is good for nerve regeneration.

In October 2014, we began searching for a hospital that could take Sharne as an out-patient for rehabilitation. We still cannot find a place.

Sharne's condition declined sharply at the beginning of 2015. We tried the B spot treatment, which is a treatment to smear nasopharynx with zinc chloride, but it was not effective for her.

By March, her condition was so bad her doctor asked one hospital to take Sharne, but this hospital did not allow Sharne to stay even though her erythrocyte sedimentation rate was greater than 60 (it had been around 30 before). Later in March 2015, the respiratory distress which Sharne had experienced during the first two years after Cervarix injection, returned. She was sent to a hospital by an ambulance but sent home without treatment.

In April, I as a parent thought that she may not survive. I visited nearly 50 hospitals. Sometimes I could not even talk to a doctor. They just sent me back home. I was exhausted. I decided for the first time I should give up and accept her fate.

There seemed to be no doctors in Japan trying to help the children who were suffering in front of them. No one seemed prepared to try and treat conditions for which there was no easy diagnosis. We used to have good old ethics and morals. We used to share other people's pain.

I remember watching a TV documentary where a girl injured by the HPV vaccine said, "I found out that nobody helps me." I understood exactly how she felt and surrendered.

When I gave up, my husband seemed more determined to help Sharne. He telephoned the hospital that gave Sharne the IAPP. Although the hospital had turned down multiple requests from me, they agreed to my husband's strong request this time.

We returned to the hospital hoping another IAPP treatment would improve Sharne's condition only to discover she was too weak to endure the treatment. In her current condition, there was a high probability of her developing heart failure. They proposed a blood transfusion, but my daughter refused it. We decided to go home this time and come back after Sharne regained some physical strength.

This was the only hospital we found in Japan that accepted all patients equally and tried to help the people who were suffering. Because this was the only hospital in Japan that gave IAPP treatments to girls who had been injured by HPV vaccines, there was a long waiting list.

Sharne received IAPP in June and September 2015. Sharne did not have a lot of IgG antibodies in her body, so it took a longer time to produce them again. Thus, it took longer than normal for the outcome of the treatments to appear. When the benefits did begin to show up, they were sometimes difficult to see. However, I thought her condition improved with each treatment and the effects seemed to last longer.

In October, a doctor whom Sharne saw in April when she hit rock bottom became her primary doctor. But he refused to prescribe the steroid and the suppressant. Sharne had five asthma attacks over a period of two months. So, she started to take the suppressant. She still has asthma attacks sometimes.

There was no improvement in gait or grip strength. Malaise was still very severe. Painful muscle spasms seemed to be intensifying. Visual field constriction and visual acuity were getting worse. However, her consciousness, motivation, and mental abilities were improving. In test results, the sedimentation rate, IgE, IgD and eosinophil count were still high but beginning to decline. She still had slight fevers. In the psychological test, IQ rose for the first time but her processing speed was still decreasing. Nevertheless, her overall physical condition became somewhat stable.

Sharne had severe brain inflammation repeatedly. As of April 2017, she has been free from severe attacks since autumn 2014. Finally, I have the feeling she might have overcome the worst.

During the last three years, she received four courses of IAPP. Her grip strength usually became 2 kg immediately after IAPP and returned to 0 soon after. After her IAPP treatment in January 2017, her grip strength was 5 kg for both left and right hands and remained there when tested in April. She still has slight fevers. Her gait improved after making special shoes for correcting clubfoot. However, she still cannot walk a long distance and is unstable even with a walking stick. Her menstruation usually returned to normal period of 28 days without PMS for the first one after IAPP, but the time between menstruations gradually increases. Malaise and painful muscle spasm are gradually intensifying.

Her POTS symptoms started to alleviate after 4th IAPP therapy. Girls who are not severely affected seem to be able to maintain this state. If a girl receives IAPP immediately after the onset of symptoms, she seems to improve without receiving IAPP repeatedly. In Sharne's case the effects of IAPP lasted only one week when she received her first treatment, but the effective period gradually became longer after each subsequent treatment. She had IAPP in January this year, and in April although she still has malaise and muscle spasms, she is free from dystonia and severe involuntary movement. Her visual field constriction had been improving, but started to widen a little at the end of December 2016. Her vision is still deteriorating.

When tested for Wechsler Intelligence Scale for Children, her processing speed and motor movement are still low but other scores have improved a lot. She still has tremors all the time and sometimes has small involuntary movements and weakness of knee, but she is more stable now.

The blood sedimentation rate is around 15 to 20, IgE is 450 to 700, and 50% hemolytic complement activity (CH-50) is about 48. The neutrophil count and eosinophil count are usually within a normal value. We could not arrange for measurement of anti-ganglioside antibodies and anti-glutamate receptor antibodies.

When Sharne showed side effects from the vaccine, my husband and I thought they were due to brain inflammation. We studied, researched, and then hoped to receive an immunotherapy. However, we could not find a doctor who was willing to provide treatment. We ended up having to travel 1500 km to get to a hospital for treatments.

I think IAPP has the fewest side effects of the various types of immunotherapies available. Steroids pose a risk of osteoporosis. Immune-suppressants increase the risk of cancer. IVIG treatments need the blood of tens of thousands of people. IAPP only uses a dialysis filter (column). Any hospital with dialysis equipment can do IAPP treatments after learning the technique.

My husband, my daughter and I had firsthand experience with the effects of IAPP. Our daughter was affected more seriously by this vaccine than some other girls and it was a long time before we could start the treatments. Girls who received the treatment early now live independently and have progressed to further education, which gave us a huge hope. We believe that our daughter can do the same in future. We hope that this treatment option spreads worldwide, so people who suffer from the side effects of HPV vaccines can recover sooner.

Sharne graduated from a junior high school, but she cannot start a senior high school yet. We had saved money for her education, but the money was spent on the cost of medical treatments. Part of the expensive treatment fee is paid from the tax collected from people in Japan. Many girls and women who are injured after HPV vaccines will be supported by the tax in future instead of contributing to it.

Is it not common sense that companies should be responsible for any damage caused by the products they manufacture? There are so many injuries after injecting HPV vaccines. I wished that they had researched possible side effects and tested all data for supporting prevention of cancer before marketing and shipping these vaccines. I cannot understand why they are not being held accountable for what they have done.

I believe in the words given by a fortune-telling lady that 'Sharne will be hailed as a great working woman'. I believe that she has been chosen to eliminate this tragic injustice.

CHAPTER 4

Australasia

Australia

In November 2006, Australia's Pharmaceutical Benefits Advisory Committee (PBAC) decided Gardasil was too expensive and just might not be all it was cracked up to be. So, they rejected the application for use in the national immunization schedule as well as refusing to grant Gardasil in the Pharmaceutical Benefits Scheme (PBS) subsidy program.

Health Minister, Tony Abbott, was concerned about the additional projected expenditure of $650 million over the next four years, particularly since Australia was already investing in a highly successful cervical cancer screening program that was already costing the taxpayers $60 million each year. He was well aware of the fact a recent Senate committee on gynecological cancers had just reported that cervical cancer was the only type of gynecological cancer for which the prevalence was expected to decrease despite the country's aging population.

When Health Minister Abbott made the public announcement rejecting Gardasil, he was forthright with his concerns. First and foremost, he did not believe his country should invest an additional $650 million over the next four years when they already had a safe and effective means of controlling cervical cancer. He also voiced concerns about the unproven efficacy as well as the possibility that the proposed vaccination program might result in 'an increase in cancer rates'.

Twenty-four hours later, Prime Minister John Howard decided to 'put an end to all the nonsense'. In a classic example of 'let's fix what's not broken' he sang the praises of Gardasil and issued clear orders to Minister Abbott that the immunization program should proceed with all haste. Prime Minister Howard stated, "There is no lack of desire to get this wonderful drug available and the mass immunization campaign to start as soon as possible."

Is it possible that the Prime Minister's rejection of his Health Minister's decision was influenced by the fact that Professor Ian Frazer, University of Queensland, was one of the inventors of the vaccine?

Could the Prime Minister's decision have anything to do with the fact that Professor Frazer's university owned a 6 percent global royalty on Gardasil sales and stood to gain a substantial influx of funds?[94]

So, by over-ruling the advice of the Minister of Health, Australia became one of the first four countries in the world to include HPV vaccines in their national immunization program.[95]

Australia rolled out their new HPV vaccination program in 2007 via a school-based program that initially targeted only girls. Girls ages 12-13 would receive all three doses of Gardasil in school. Those from age 14-19 could receive free doses via local providers. In 2013, the program was extended to boys and the recommended dose changed from three to two for those under the age of 15. A third dose was recommended for those who were over 15 at the time of their first injection. For anyone over the age of 20, Gardasil was available but had to be paid for privately. HPV vaccines are currently approved for use in males age 9-26 and females age 9-45.[96]

It didn't take long for problems to become apparent in the new HPV vaccination program. According to an article in *The Online Opinion,* in June 2007, four Melbourne schoolgirls were rushed to the hospital after receiving the vaccine promoted as preventing cervical cancer. Sixteen others were reported sick. One student reported being paralyzed for hours. She said, "I couldn't move at all. There were girls dropping like flies." Apparently, other schools were having similar problems.[97]

[94] Stevens, Mathew; Howard rescues Gardasil from Abbott poison pill; The Weekend Australian; 11 Nov 2006; accessed March 2019

[95] Markowitz, LE; Human papillomavirus vaccine introduction-the first five years; Vaccine; 26 Feb 2014; PMID 23199957

[96] HPV Vaccine Australia; website; accessed March 2019

Also in 2007, five schoolgirls at Sacred Heart Girls' College in suburban Melbourne, Australia, were confirmed to have taken ill after receiving an injection of Gardasil. Soon after the vaccination, twenty-six girls were seen at the campus medical clinic; five were admitted to the hospital after being injected. Two of the girls were kept in overnight in observation for dizziness; one had temporary paralysis and loss of speech.[98]

After investigating multiple cases of suspected anaphylaxis in Australia after Gardasil injections, scientists published a paper in 2008 which concluded that the estimated rate of anaphylaxis following Gardasil was "significantly higher than identified in comparable school-based delivery of other vaccines." [99]

December 2009, Dr. Ian Sutton, neurologist at St. Vincent's Hospital in Queensland, reported five cases of multiple sclerosis (MS) after Gardasil injections. All five young women had experienced the onset of symptoms within three weeks after their HPV vaccine injections.

Dr. Sutton stated, "Gardasil vaccination is not the cause of MS; whether or not it was a trigger for episodes of inflammation in the brain in these rare cases is unclear."

According to the Therapeutic Goods Administration (TGA), at the time 1476 suspected adverse reactions to Gardasil had already been reported. A spokesman for the regulatory agency stated, "The TGA is also aware of a small number of cases in which neurological symptoms, similar to those experienced in patients with a demyelinating disorder such as multiple sclerosis, have been reported shortly after HPV (human papillomavirus vaccination)."[100]

By March 2011, *Medical News Today* reported almost a quarter of Australian girls were 'not taking advantage' of Gardasil despite it being available free of charge. The article blamed the problem on 'an alarming lack of knowledge'.[101]

---

[97] Klein, Renata; Tankard-Reist, Melinda; Gardasil: we must not ignore the risks; Online Opinion; 1 June 2007; accessed March 2019

[98] Dr. Tenpenny, Sherri; Gardasil Dangers Starting to Emerge; NewsWithViews.com; 24 May 2007; accessed March 2019

[99] Julia M.L. Brotherton, MD MPH, et al; Anaphylaxis following quadrivalent human papillomavirus vaccination; 9 Sept 2008; PMID 18762618

[100] Labi, Sharon; Gardasil linked to MS symptoms; originally published in *The Courier Mail*; 13 Dec 2009; available on SaneVax.org

[101] Staff Writer; Quarter of Girls Missing Out on Life-Saving Vaccine: New

In 2012, the Australian media began to quote a recently published article suggesting HPV vaccine use should be extended to boys in order to provide useful insights for all countries.

According to one report, multiple researchers decided that the experiences and data gained from countries where gender-equal HPV vaccination was instituted would provide essential information to further understand the impact of dual-sex HPV vaccination programs.

Kirby Institute Sexual Health Program head Professor Basil Donovan said, "Australia is the best case study because we're so far ahead of every other country in the world in immunizing girls."[102]

By the end of June 2013, Australia's database of adverse event notifications had recorded over 1991 suspected side effects following the 'cervical cancer' vaccine.[103]

Later the same year, Dr. Deidre Little presented a case study detailing new onset of menstrual disturbance and oligo-menorrhea with symptoms beginning four months after one of her patients received Gardasil. The symptoms proceeded to premature ovarian failure over the next twenty-four months. Prior to receiving Gardasil her patient had been a healthy 16-year-old girl.[104] In 2014, Dr. Little published a paper outlining the case studies of three girls, ages 16, 16, and 18 who had all experienced the onset of ovarian decline after Gardasil injections.[105]

In spite of all the controversy surrounding HPV vaccines, or perhaps because of it, the Australian government announced a new 'no jab, no pay' measure. From 1 January 2016 on, children of all ages must be up to date with their immunizations or lose eligibility for their annual Child

---

Website Aims to Reverse Trend, Australia; Medical News Today; 10 March 2011; accessed March 2019

[102] Staff Writers; Male HPV Vaccination Would Help the World; Research; Star Observer; 3 April 2012; accessed March 2019

[103] Klein, Renata; Lobato, Helen; Australia must also caution on Gardasil; Online Opinion; 28 June 2013; accessed March 2019

[104] Little, Deidre, MMBS DRANZCOG, FACRRM; human Papillomavirus vaccine and the Ovary: The Need for Research; presentation at the 18th World Congress on Controversies in Obstetrics, Gynecology, and Infertility; Oct 2013; print version available on SaneVax.org

[105] Little, DT, Ward, HR; Adolescent Premature Ovarian insufficiency Following Human Papillomavirus Vaccination: A Case Series Seen in General Practice; Journal of Investigative Medicine High Impact Case Reports; 28 Oct 2014; PMID 26425627

Care Benefit (CCB) and Child Care Rebate (CCR) financial supplements. Exceptions would only be granted for medical reasons.[106] Media reports suggested around 10,000 families would lose eligibility for payments in 2016-17 as a result of the new policy. Many more were expected to ensure their children, including teens, were up-to-date with their childhood immunizations in order to survive financially.

One has to ask what do such draconian measures cost the families of Australia, not only financially, but emotionally?

Are outcomes like those in the next few pages to be considered acceptable collateral damage in the quest for optimum vaccine uptake?

---

[106] Klapdor, Michael; Grove, Alex; 'No Jab, No Pay' and other immunization measures; Parliament of Australia Budget Review; 2015-16; accessed March 2019

Why didn't someone warn us?

By Jenny from Australia

Jemma, my first born beautiful, gorgeous bundle of joy was growing into a happy, vibrant, bubbly child. We certainly endured numerous challenging times because my happy, fun-loving, noisy child always had plenty of energy to burn and such a strong personality.

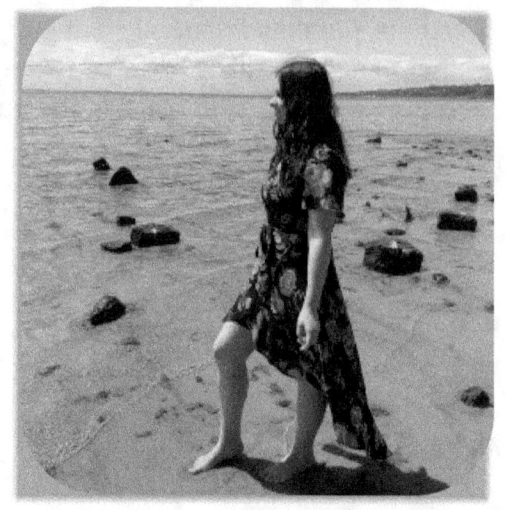

As Jemma grew, she absolutely loved socializing with her peers. Jemma's first interest was dancing. I enrolled Jemma into dance lessons at the age of 5-years-old. She exhibited a natural ability from the beginning. She was extremely flexible and I often would see her doing the splits, cartwheels and bridges. Jemma continued to dance right through her primary school years. When she entered grade 6, she also became interested in horse-riding. So, we added riding lessons to her schedule and eventually intended to buy her a horse.

Jemma was enrolled to start her secondary schooling in 2014. The catholic school we had chosen for her to attend had recently expanded their campus. She was about to begin the new school year in a brand-new portion of the school's three campuses. Jemma was 12-years-old and had always considered herself quite confident. However, the nerves did kick in a bit while anticipating starting the year in a new school.

Jemma settled in well meeting new people and working out her new schedule. Jemma enjoyed her first term which was approximately ten weeks. During this term we received a letter along with a consent form to fill out for Jemma to receive the HPV Vaccine and Varicella (chicken pox) vaccine.

I read the immunization brochure and I thought, "Yes, I want to protect my daughter against cervical cancer."

However I was aware it was a new vaccine and I wasn't 100% convinced. I discussed this with my husband and he basically said, "We didn't have this when we were young, and we were all fine." With his second breath he said, "What a load of shit!"

I replied, "No, I think this is a good idea and I want to protect Jemma."

After all, Jemma had been fully vaccinated by the recommendations from the Australian immunization government guidelines to date.

Even so, I thought it would be best to do some research. However I failed to follow this through. I trusted our health system. I also started thinking about my niece who had it. She was fine, so that sealed my decision. I decided that Jemma would have this vaccine. I wanted to give her the best protection I could and I was under the assumption it would protect her against cervical cancer. However I wanted her to have it done at our doctor's office so I could be there to support her.

Looking back now, my sister says her daughter was very fatigued the year she received Gardasil, but they basically put it down to the added pressures of starting secondary school.

Jemma's first shot was given in February 2014. She complained of a very heavy sore arm, but I didn't think much of it. After all, a little soreness is expected after most vaccines.

Jemma had her second shot on Thursday 24th April. Three days later, during our Sunday lunch, life began to tumble into despair. We were at a racetrack where my son was racing a quarter midget and Jemma was sitting in the car. The temperature was around 19°C (66°F). Jemma complained of dizziness, not feeling well, and a sudden headache. I blamed her for sitting in the warm car and not drinking enough water.

We left approximately a few hours later and, on the way home I decided to give her a Panadol. However after taking it, she still had a headache. I thought this was extremely unusual. Any other time I had given her Panadol it would relieve her. That evening she still wasn't feeling well and was quite fatigued.

By the next day, she was still feeling fatigued and still had the headache. I started to think, "Did the HPV vaccine play a role?" I immediately rang the doctor and made an appointment.

During this appointment, my doctor believed she was having an adverse reaction to the vaccine and said her headache will disappear in two weeks, then referred us to a chiropractor.

On consultation with our chiropractor, we were advised Jemma was suffering from 'a rare highly debilitating condition of vaccine-injury syndrome.' She told us symptoms vary from patient to patient. However in Jemma's case she is suffering constant, unremitting headaches, constant fatigue, difficulty concentrating, pain in her arms and legs, as well as weakness of limbs, bowel sensitivity and some visual disturbances.

Two weeks later the headache was still there so I went back to our doctor. He suggested Jemma take Periactin 4mg. I wasn't keen to put her on this however I did for one week only. After reading the side effects I decided to stop as I was too frightened.

Our doctor had also referred us to see a pediatrician who said he had never seen a patient with such protracted symptoms. He was at a loss as how to help Jemma other than run some blood tests and refer us to the Royal Melbourne Children's Hospital. I had already been in contact with the hospital because my GP had reported her injury to TGA. I found them to be of not much help. The hospital had simply suggested her headaches were related to her eyes and that I should get her eyes tested. I did have her eyes tested however I knew this was not the cause.

When the blood test results came back, they had detected the presence of Epstein Barr virus and high white cells and neutrophils. I felt lost. My daughter was feeling so sick and no one seemed to know how to help her. It was extremely frustrating to feel like there was nowhere to turn.

In a desperate attempt to find help and answers for Jemma, I started to search the internet trying to find doctors who had experience dealing with vaccine injuries. I came across a USA doctor treating Gardasil-injured children. I had arranged for a Skype session with him. This doctor had incredible knowledge regarding what HPV vaccines were doing to certain individuals. He was kind, caring and compassionate and I was about to order the tests he recommended.

That same week, I happened to visit my local dentist for treatment and I mentioned how my daughter become ill after the HPV vaccine. The dental nurse said she knew of someone's daughter who was so seriously injured after Gardasil that she almost died. Maybe this lady could help us.

I contacted this lady and after speaking with her, I realized I wasn't alone. Thousands of families worldwide were also suffering. She suggested I join a Facebook group to connect with other families damaged after HPV vaccinations. I was utterly GOBSMACKED and NUMB at how so many were suffering the exact same symptoms as my daughter. I could hardly believe so many had died. It made me physically sick to know how many were suffering. I felt utterly helpless. I didn't know how to help my own daughter, much less be able to do anything for all of the others.

I began to follow the same healing path of the lady that I met through my dentist. I cancelled my appointments with the USA doctor as I thought it would be much easier seeing someone in my own country to try and heal Jemma. I made an appointment with this neuro-trainer, kinesiologist, and naturopath. However the earliest available appointment was in 4 weeks, so I decided to see a local naturopath while waiting for her. This naturopath started her on a detox, used acupuncture, and supplements. She also did a hair analysis test that showed toxic substance exposure and metal contaminants. We began changing her diet to gluten free, dairy free, and no sugar. We started buying all organic fruit and vegetables along with all-natural products for skin care and home use.

I also took the advice of several others in our Facebook support groups because we shared such similar experiences. These families offered unbelievable support and a wealth of knowledge. We talked about what worked as well as what didn't work. We compared the progress our daughters were making along with their setbacks. Simply talking to people who understood was a great source of comfort and support.

For instance, there was one mother in Ireland, Kiva Murphy, with whom I spoke regularly. I could almost say her daughter was Jemma's twin. They shared identical symptoms. We spoke often, continually sharing our healing methods and progress reports. We had so much in common.

In spite of all the moral support, I still spent a lot of time riddled with guilt. I could not seem to forgive myself for allowing my daughter to be injected with Gardasil when I had so many unanswered questions. Once

I started to research further, I became extremely angry. To this day, I cannot comprehend how HPV vaccines are still on the market.

I found out about Dr. Deirdre Little's discovery and watched her YouTube video where she talked about diagnosing three young girls with premature ovarian failure after their Gardasil jabs. I believe now she has reported seven cases. She followed up with extensive research subsequently published her findings in the BMJ. Apparently, the drug company MERCK forgot to do studies on the ovaries. I was totally stunned and shocked!

I became very concerned about Jemma's hormones, so I contacted Dr. Little. She was incredibly helpful and recommended that when Jemma turned 14 we needed to test her hormones. I had taken Dr. Little's peer reviewed article to my Doctor because he didn't believe infertility could be a possible outcome. I think the peer-reviewed published paper took him by surprise. His response was, "Well, it's a fairly new vaccine and we don't know enough about it."

I felt outraged that my daughter had basically been subjected to being a guinea pig for this pointless vaccine! I spent many nights crying myself to sleep, asking myself, "Why is this happening, why?" I was overcome with such unbearable sadness. I could not stop grieving for my once happy healthy child who was now so sick. I watched her friends meeting all their milestones while Jemma fought hard to overcome her health ailments. This continually ripped at my heart strings. I would often say, "Why us?"

Jemma was suffering terribly. With each passing day it became worse. Her headaches were so intense, she felt her head was going to explode. She was constantly holding her head saying, "My head is so sore!"

This was repeated to me up to 20 times a day. She also started experiencing 20-second silent seizures. At the time, I had no idea what was happening. She would simply stop moving, her face frozen and staring at me while her mouth slightly moved to a smiling position. This went on for approximately two months. At the same time, Jemma became sensitive to noise and light, her heart would frequently beat rapidly and her eyes felt like they couldn't open.

I thought, "Oh my goodness she has been poisoned by this vaccine that was supposedly meant to protect her."

Once again, I became extremely angry! How could this possibly happen?

During the next two months, more new symptoms appeared. She began to experience tingling and numbness in her legs, bottom and feet, her ears started to ring, abdominal pain and vomiting became extreme. Jemma found the only way to get comfortable at night was to sleep upright because she had to endure tremendous pain in her abdomen when lying down. Her level of fatigue was extremely high.

One day, I found Jemma on the bathroom floor in a fetal position suffering extreme abdominal pain along with vomiting. It was horrific to witness! We called the ambulance immediately. The doctor at the hospital referred us to a pediatric gastroenterology specialist who didn't believe the HPV vaccine could have caused Jemma's issues.

However, when the doctor left, a nurse whispered to me, "I'm so sorry this has happened to your daughter."

She went on to say she had researched this vaccine and opted out of giving it to her daughters.

Ultimately, the pediatric gastroenterology specialist said at the outset that Jemma did not have Crohn's disease and suggested she had fructose malabsorption. He believed her headaches and extreme fatigue coincided with receiving the HPV vaccine. Laboratory tests demonstrated neutrophilia. He suggested an MRI if her neurologic symptoms persisted.

Jemma's constant headaches remained persistent with a constant sore throat (She would describe it like having a bubble or lump in her throat) along with muscle aches in her upper arms and legs. Her body temperature was often cold and she continued feeling dizzy. It became increasingly difficult for her to concentrate. She found it very difficult to sleep. I would frequently have to lie beside her massaging her head as it was so painful in order to help her get to sleep.

In July 2014, Jemma began dropping things, sometimes the lightest items like paper. She started to experience twitching; then she complained of her hips aching; then her legs collapsed underneath her. She barely could walk. I was at a loss. I felt like no health professional knew how to help. This continued for three weeks, so I decided to get some crutches to help her. Jemma regained her ability to walk, however she was very weak. It was difficult for her to walk short distances. Stairs or up hills were impossible.

We started on reflexology and foot spas. This eased her pain temporarily. Jemma continued losing the ability to walk at unpredictable times. She often described her legs as feeling dead. This went on for months.

I also reached out to a USA researcher who was offering information to several families with Gardasil injured children. He suggested Jemma could be suffering from Bartonella, a co-infection to Lyme. Apparently, he believed both infections can remain dormant in a person's body until activated by Gardasil vaccinations. I tried to suggest this possibility to her health practitioners, but they dismissed it because they didn't believe Bartonella existed in Australia. Her doctor diagnosed her with a neurological disorder.

Jemma had three months off school. We tried to get her back for at least two hours a day with several days in between. This went on for the next 6 months. During that time, she would constantly text me saying she felt sick. Jemma was fortunate enough to have two teachers who were extremely caring and understanding of her illness.

However, one teacher we came across wasn't so understanding and made comments to her regarding her poor attendance. I picked Jemma up one day and she was so upset she was shaking. During her entire school career, she had never experienced this type of distress from a teacher's words. When Jemma found the work too hard, because it felt like her brain was on fire and foggy, this teacher just kept telling her, she COULD. Jemma felt she was constantly dismissing her health conditions. This teacher also kept telling Jemma she needed to attend more days at school.

I approached this teacher in a nice way, and said, "Please do not decide when Jemma should or shouldn't be at school. We are working closely with her medical and holistic practitioners."

Then, I burst into tears. I just couldn't cope with the extra drama. The principal called my husband and I in for a meeting and I got the impression this teacher had most likely exaggerated what I had said. In spite of this, we were able to discuss what could be done to accommodate Jemma's learning needs. I began to realize how difficult it is for parents who have a child out of mainstream with learning difficulties or suffering from a chronic illness. I also realized it was in my best interest to go straight to the principal whenever I had a problem.

Jemma's life continued to tumble downhill. Most of the time she wouldn't leave our home. On rare occasions, she tried to visit friends or have sleepovers. But, I was always called to come and get her because the pain made it too difficult to be around people.

We continued taking Jemma to the neuro-trainer kinesiologist who had been recommended by our dental nurse, whose daughter also suffered terribly. I was so desperate for answers, I was relentless in my research. I wanted her healed.

I had also come across a health clinic for people suffering chronic fatigue, so we began a 12-week program there. Her pain and fatigue continued, so we also began seeing a physiotherapist to help with her leg pain.

On the advice from a friend who had been suffering wrist pain that disappeared after being treated by a certain practitioner, we decided to see the same acupuncture specialist. I was open to any referrals from friends. I just wanted my daughter to get better. We continued treatment for approximately eight to ten weeks. Jemma would have temporary relief from her pain, however it still continued.

We also continued to have regular chiropractic treatments along with cupping and infrared saunas.

By November, I told my doctor I was concerned with her head pain and asked for an MRI. The results came back with 'normal intracranial appearance right-sided sinus mucosal disease.'

The principal sent us a letter concerned about how much school Jemma has missed. He suggested we repeat year 7 over a two-year period. I spoke with health professionals and was advised not to accept this offer considering she was still suffering. Their opinion was forcing her to repeat year 7 would negatively affect her socially. So, Jemma went into year 8 despite having missed so much school.

Jemma began to get unusual marks on her body which looked like scratches or stretch marks. Health professionals were saying they were stretch marks. I wasn't totally convinced as she wasn't a large girl and the marks changed color from red to deep purple.

By this time, I was connected with thousands of other families worldwide through Facebook so I started asking questions and sending photos of her marks. Several families believed she had Bartonella.

A few days later, I was walking out of her school and bumped into another mother who asked how Jemma was. I explained all of her symptoms and she immediately told me she knew someone who was suffering similar symptoms and had been diagnosed with Lyme and co-infections. She suggested we see a Lyme literate medical doctor, something quite rare in Australia. We did find someone and I made an appointment to see him in May 2015. He clinically diagnosed Jemma with Bartonella and suggested we run some blood tests. He also said we may need to send her blood samples overseas to Igenex Lab in the United States because they have more accurate testing for Lyme and co-infections. He indicated the tests done in Australia generally give a false negative reading as the bacteria is very clever at hiding. We ended up sending her blood samples to Igenex Lab and they came back positive to Lyme and six co-infections.

This doctor wanted to treat her with extensive antibiotics however I was very hesitant to start this type of treatment. Jemma was already allergic to antibiotics. I was concerned about stripping her gut bacteria and didn't like the list of potential side effects. The doctor said there were other ways to treat Lyme, so we ended up putting her on an herbal protocol where she would be taking up to 35 supplements and herbs a day.

In this doctor's opinion Jemma was suffering from symptoms of multi-system infectious disease syndrome which appears to have occurred as a result of the Gardasil injections for the human papilloma virus. He believed the jabs caused a number of low-grade bacterial infections which her immune system had previously had under control to become reactivated. As a result, Jemma suffered from chronic tiredness, headaches, painful muscles (fibromyalgia), and episodes of cardiac palpitations, breathlessness, and numbness in some areas of her body and limited stamina which explained her inability to walk for sustained periods.

As it turned out, our doctor was in contact with a Professor in Germany who had diagnosed over 100 Irish girls all with Lyme and co-infections after having the HPV vaccine. In the Professor's opinion, Gardasil could reactivate Borrelia, Bartonella, Chlamydia pn, and Mycoplasma pn, EBV, CMV, HSV1, HSV2, and Coxsackie. Jemma had been diagnosed with three from this list (Borrelia, Bartonella and EBV).

At this point, we decided to pull Jemma out of school. Some weeks she could only attend school for 2 hours. We were paying private school fees for no service because Jemma was too sick to attend. We decided to enroll her in homeschool with limited subjects. She often finds even this limited schedule difficult.

The neuro-trainer we were seeing was an hour's drive for us so she suggested we see a colleague she had trained that was closer to us. That way, we could have more frequent appointments as we were only able to see her once a month when she flew in to treat the patients at her clinic. We decided to start a 10-week program with the colleague she recommended and continue our once a month treatments with her.

Jemma began to listen to music and sing, so I encouraged her to begin guitar lessons. Jemma started and continued for 12 weeks. However in the end, she found it too hard to concentrate and gave up.

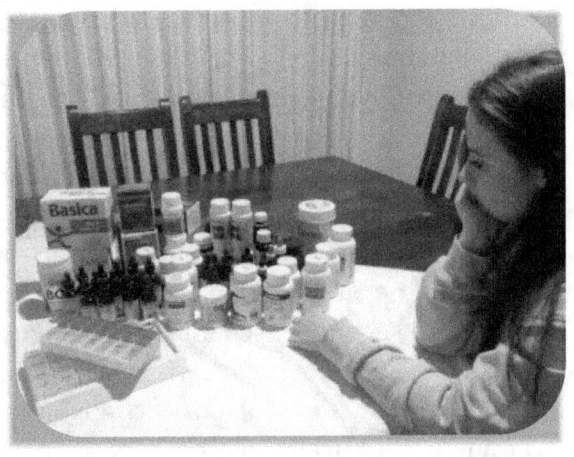

Jemma has connected with numerous teenagers from other countries through Facebook and social media. I keep a close eye on this though I am happy for her to be able to interact with others her age. Some would ask why she wasn't in school. When she felt comfortable, she would share her experiences.

Jemma is fortunate enough to still have some close friends from her school who stay in contact with her. She met a girl in student programs, a program set up for children with special learning difficulties. This particular girl was dealing with a diagnosis of brain cancer when Jemma met her. She is now in remission. They became very close friends while dealing with their respective chronic illnesses and are great company for each other to this day.

Jemma and I met up with another injured girl and her mother when she flew into Melbourne for treatment. It brought such comfort to the girls and me just to be there and support one another.

We continued seeing the neuro-trainer once every month. Meanwhile, the more research I did the more frustrated I got at how this could be happening. As a parent, I felt I wasn't given enough information to make an informed decision. I strongly believe every patient deserves to be given the complete vaccine insert before they are asked whether or not to be injected with an HPV vaccine.

In September 2015, I decided to send a letter to the Archbishop of Melbourne and the Catholic Education Office voicing my concerns surrounding Gardasil. I attached several peer reviewed articles to each letter.

The Archbishop replied saying thank you for taking the time to express my concerns about the HPV vaccine and that he was grateful for the information I provided him. He said he would share the information with the director of education so all may be alerted to what is happening.

I also received a letter back from the Catholic Education Department stating he acknowledged the impact our family has experienced and appreciated me taking the time to raise this matter with him. He basically said the Australian Government introduced this vaccine in 2007 as part of a national school-based vaccination initiative. He went on to say the HPV vaccine is administered via arrangements with local councils to secondary school students aged 12-13 years to protect them against a range of cancers and diseases caused by the human papillomavirus. He sent links to government sites regarding the HPV vaccine and basically said parents were well informed. I believe this is not the case because every parent deserves to read the vaccine insert before making a decision.

In November, I attended a seminar on functional neurology which in my understanding examines disorders of the nervous system. I decided to start Jemma on treatments using this type of therapy. During the initial physical examination, Jemma demonstrated right-hand side functional hemispheric signs including pyramidal weakness, increased pain sensation and tone in the anterior compartment in the upper limb, palatal weakness and percussion myotonia. Jemma showed signs of functional left weakness, foot tapping and dysdiadochokinesia at the shoulder and elbow. All of these symptoms are included in Fukuda's 1994 description of CFS. There was no evidence of POTS.

Jemma's EEG/Loreta analysis showed hypo-activation in the front parietal cortex in all ranges. There is pan cortical hypo-activation present in the High Beta, Gamma and High Gamma frequencies with exception of hyper-activation in the right temporal cortex and around Fz. There is hyper-activation also present in the right occipital cortex.

Her treatment schedule was three visits per week over a 12-week period. We drove an hour up and back to each appointment. We also met another family affected after Gardasil having the same treatment as Jemma.

Jemma's second EEG scan after 12 weeks demonstrated hypo-activation in the left temporal cortex in all frequencies excluding Delta. There was hypo-activation present in the central cortex in all Gamma,

Beta 3 and High Beta frequencies. Hypo-activation can also be visualized in the right front-temporal region in all Alpha, and High Gamma frequencies. Hyper-activation was present in the central region of Theta, Alpha 2 and Beta 1 frequencies. A focal area of hyper-activation could be visualized over F8 in all Beta and all Gamma frequencies, excluding High Gamma. Alpha and Alpha 1 frequencies demonstrate hyper-activation in the left occipital region over O1. Hyper-activation was also demonstrated in the frontal region of Delta frequency, and focally over Fz in the High Gamma frequency. Abnormal activity noticed in both eyes open and eyes closed scans.

Upon review abnormal activity was also seen in scans from 3/12/2015. Upon visual inspection of raw data trace an increase in frequency was seen at the T8 electrode throughout the recording. The high T3 could be artefact from a hyperactive temporalis muscle or TMJ. My understanding was she was damaged in the peripheral sensory.

Sadly Jemma couldn't continue this treatment as the Melbourne Clinic was closing down, so we would have had to travel interstate to the other clinics to receive this treatment.

When Jemma turned 14, I decided to have her hormones checked as Dr. Little had suggested. Our doctor ordered the tests which Dr. Little suggested should be done. Jemma's results came back with extremely high prolactin so my doctor ordered her to have an MRI. The results of this MRI showed her pituitary was normal in size. The results also showed a lesion in the left cerebrum extending from lateral ventricle to the vertex of the cortex/subcortical region which was somewhat band-like and raises the possibility of type two focal cortical dysplasia sign.

We decided to make an appointment to see a pediatric neurologist whom I found to be blunt, arrogant and very black and white. I told him my daughter had been diagnosed with Lyme and co-infections. He arrogantly replied, "I will speak to you in two years." He wasn't open to speaking about the previous diagnosis at all.

Then he said, "Your daughter has no life. It's like having a broken bone, the plaster comes off and you have to rehabilitate it back."

To be honest I found him to have no bedside manners at all. I got the impression he thought he had an incredibly high status by virtue of being 'educated.' I remained composed and calm. He told me the MRI demonstrated a lesion in the left cerebrum that is concerning because of possible cortical dysplasia.

Jemma was still experiencing poor sleep hygiene, going to sleep between midnight to 4am and waking between 10am to 11am. He recommended better sleep hygiene and asked her to keep a headache diary. I basically said she has a constant headache. He referred us to a modified rehabilitation program so she could get back to school as soon as possible. He believed her inability to attend school was causing social disruption. He also said we need to follow up on the MRI as I left his office.

I wasn't satisfied with his advice and refused his rehabilitation program. We continued Jemma's neuro-training every two months as our neuro-trainer lived interstate and now flew down every two months instead of each month.

I approached my local MP who wrote a letter to the Minster of Health in February 2016 on my behalf. The response he received was similar to others. It basically outlined the procedure of vaccines here in Australia and stressed that they are thoroughly tested for safety and efficacy. The letter went on to say that in development, vaccines are rigorously tested on thousands of people in progressively larger clinical trials. It also stressed that vaccines are not administered in Australia until they have been approved for use by the therapeutic goods administration to ensure they meet safety guidelines, and are evaluated to ensure they are effective, comply with strict manufacturing and production standards, and have a good safety record.

Meanwhile, Jemma was still having serious symptoms. Every day she would wake saying she felt sick. We decided to visit another doctor who suggested running further blood tests. Her CD3 Mature T, CD4 Helper T, CD56 B Cell were high, so this doctor decided to start IV treatments. We started this IV treatment giving her normal saline infusion, inj. B 2ml, inj. magnesium sulphate 5ml, inj. trace elements 5ml and inj. vitamin C <=15g (30g/100ml), but on the third visit the nurse hit a tendon and Jemma refused to go back. The pain was horrible for her.

By now, Jemma was overwhelmed and sick of seeing doctors and health practitioners. She kept saying, "No one is helping me get better."

I spent numerous hours saying, "I will never give up on healing you. I know we have seen so many health practitioners, but you are improving slowly."

I felt her health was like an onion: we were slowly, very slowly peeling the layers off and she was recovering. I was determined to heal Jemma and desperate for her health to return to normal again.

Jemma continued to complain of pain in her left ovary, so we had a pelvic ultrasound. This report showed possible polycystic ovaries. We were referred to a further ultrasound with a health practitioner who had more in-depth experience. She believed the ultrasound she did was fine although questions still pop up in the back of my head from time to time because Jemma still experiences pain on one of her ovaries. Why were the results of the first ultrasound suspecting polycystic ovaries and the second one fine?

In May 2017, I decided to write another letter, this time to the new health minister. He acknowledged the distressing impact Gardasil had on our family and explained the previous health minister had already addressed my concerns. He advised me there had been no new information identified which would change the safety profile of Gardasil. I just felt helpless. I felt ignored when all I, and other parents in similar situations, wanted was for our girls and boys to have the proper care. We were so tired of having to visit numerous health professionals seeking answers.

In August 2017, I attended the screenings of the Vaxxed Documentary. This gave me an opportunity to share our story with Polly Tommey and raise further awareness. I wanted parents to know how important it is to DO their own RESEARCH.

Around this time, I got speaking with a lovely lady whose daughter suffered terribly from Lyme. Her daughter had had no vaccines. At first, they did not know why her daughter was ill, but eventually found out it was Lyme and travelled to the USA for treatment. After coming back to Australia, they sought help through a health practitioner who continued to help her daughter recover.

I was still concerned about Jemma's hormones, so I was open to seeing her to just see if she could help Jemma. She advised us to go on supplements that might help Jemma. We started and Jemma's head pain began to ease even further. We also tested her MTHFR Gene Mutation and discovered she had the MTHFR (C677T) Heterozygous. We did another test on her hormones through a saliva sample because Jemma was too frightened to have blood taken after her bad experience with the IV's. The results showed Jemma had triple the amount of estrogen she should have so we started her on DIM supplement to reduce this. We continued to see this practitioner for the next 6 months.

However, Jemma was so sick of taking supplements as this has been her life for the last three years.

We continued to see our neuro-trainer every two months. Jemma truly looked forward to these visits because she felt lighter and could think more clearly after her appointments.

In August 2018, Sacrificial Virgins Documentary was screened again, this time in Melbourne. I also spoke at this showing and shared our story. I found the night to be extremely overwhelming and hard to handle at times. Our wounds were still raw. Talking about our story forced me to re-live the hell I had experienced while trying to help Jemma recover.

I wrote another letter to our health minister trying to arrange a time to meet. His response was to refer us to the Royal Children's Hospital to seek help. He also gave me a personal e-mail to reach out to the immunization department. I sent an e-mail to arrange an appointment to meet in person, however I'm yet to receive a response.

In August 2018, I decided Jemma needed to have a genetic DNA test. Maybe it would disclose something that would give us some insights to help further improve her health. It took approximately 3 hours to go through the procedure. I was given a 98-page explanation of the results. This has given us an understanding of how her body functions and some potential directions to improve her level of healing.

I had also sought advice and opinions from four other practitioners, however we decided not to continue their treatment protocols as I wasn't convinced they would help Jemma. We were already doing very similar treatments. For instance, one protocol was going to cost us an astounding $28,000 for a three month treatment protocol involving vitamin and mineral testing, food sensitivity test/diet, bioenergetic functional re-balancing, organs test: detox, organs test parasites, bacteria, fungus, and viruses, emotional healing, oxidative therapy medical ozone: as MAH major autohemotherapy, minor AH (auto immunotherapy), UBI: ultraviolet light, blood irradiation, high dose vitamin C, antibiotic/antifungal/antiparasitic therapies, insulin targeted low-dose therapy, and enzyme therapy, DMSO and hyperthermia I. We couldn't justify this cost. Even so, over the last five years we have spent a huge amount to recover Jemma.

In December 2018, we did a follow up MRI and were happy to discover the lesion on the left side of her cerebrum had dissolved.

Jemma was still experiencing pain around her heart, so we did an ultrasound which came back clear. She still has a rapid heartbeat, however we believe this can be managed.

Jemma appears to have a lump on her neck. We made an appointment to see what this was, but the results were normal. Jemma found it hard to understand as she was still experiencing unexplained pain. I believe it is inflammation and I continue to explain to Jemma to eat very clean.

We are now in 2019, I would say Jemma is 80% recovered. She still has lingering health issues, however she manages them very well. I can only hope one day her neurological disorder disappears. Jemma still has problems reading. At any given time, she has a limit of reading four pages then her headaches become worse. Jemma basically missed out on her secondary school education and all of the typical social activities teenagers normally enjoy.

Now that Jemma has recovered most of her previous abilities, she can finally begin to look at life in a much more positive way. Jemma has shown a great interest in caring for the elderly. She started volunteering in an Aged Care Facility. We are all extremely grateful to this organization for giving her an opportunity in spite of knowing her health history. Jemma feels this environment is a happy, positive one with numerous workers helping and guiding her. Working here has given her a purpose for living. The well-being officer has said she will look at employing her on a casual or part-time basis in the future.

We just enrolled her in a course for aged care. With continued assistance from others, I think she has the ability to complete the course. Life for Jemma is finally looking good with a promising future in front of her.

I will always wonder what life would have been like for Jemma if this mess had never happened. What would her school life have been like? What kind of future would she have had without Gardasil? What kind of woman would she have been without all of the trauma she endured over the last few years? There are so many questions I will never have answers for.

I suspect these questions will always haunt me, but I know it's time to move forward with a positive outlook. We have to put this all behind us. I know we can still build a bright future.

Nevertheless, I just can't stop thinking of all the new families being damaged by HPV vaccines. Because of them, I will never stop sharing our story. I will never stop providing information to parents so they can make a fully informed decision. I wish someone would have done this for us.

Throughout this journey I have learnt to lean on numerous people. Some were very understanding and others weren't so much. However, I knew who and where I could get support from. I learnt to discuss Jemma's health issues with people who I felt never judged us. After two years, Jemma's chronic illness became an invisible one that is very hard to explain to some people as she looked fine although she felt so sick under her smile. She is incredible with such a strong outlook to those that didn't support her. However, we were extremely fortunate to have met the ones who did. They helped me get through this nightmare. I will be forever grateful to these people.

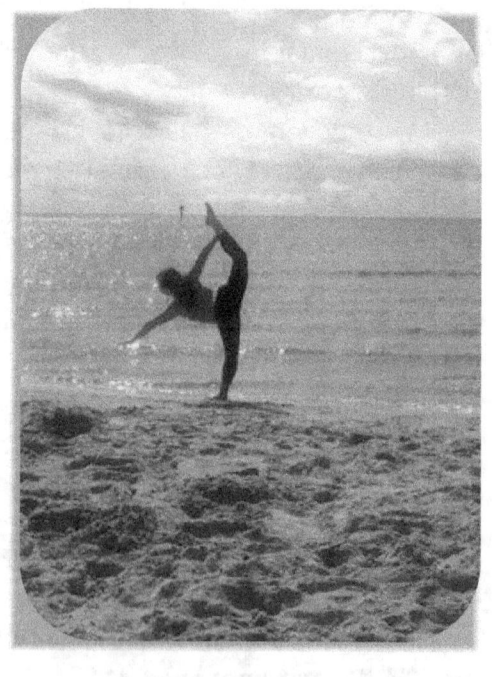

I will continue to meet and support the numerous new families who are forced to deal with the unintended consequences of HPV vaccine injections. I will continue to share our treatment protocols with others hoping they will help others heal.

Looking back, I am not exactly sure how we survived the first two years. They were by far the most difficult. Our lives rapidly became extremely stressful. Our family's life changed in so many ways. Simple walks or simple outings became difficult, sometimes impossible. Our family was compromised beyond belief. Those years crippled us financially, mentally, and emotionally. We are pleased to say we came out the other end.

I would never wish for any family, or child, to experience what we endured.

I'm so grateful we still have Jemma with us. I am glad we had the opportunity to help her heal and recover. It breaks my heart to know some families don't get this chance.

I will forever be grateful to Freda Birrell and Norma Erickson for their continuous support through the most difficult challenge of my life recovering my daughter. I felt extremely privileged to meet Norma and I hope one day I meet Freda. Their endless support and guidance has been phenomenal. They both have an incredible wealth of knowledge, not to mention unconditional empathy, kindness and compassion towards the suffering amongst so many families worldwide.

Medical and scientific experts from around the world are revealing multiple concerns regarding HPV vaccines and vaccination programs. The stories shared by families worldwide are nothing short of shocking.

I will never understand how HPV vaccines can possibly remain on the market with all of the controversy surrounding their use. How can such carnage be ignored?

Hunter Smith - HPV vaccine injury.

By Ashlea Smith, Sunshine Coast, Australia

Hunter 15, is our third child and only son. He has two older sisters, Tahlia 18 and Sophie 17. Our family resides at the beautiful Sunshine Coast, about one hour north of Brisbane, on the east coast of Australia. All of our children have led very active lives and are happy, healthy and well-rounded teenagers.

Hunter was awarded his Black belt in Karate at 12 and his second Dan at 13. He has a natural ability with both swimming and running and enjoys both. At the beginning of the year he had commenced sessions at Core-Strength Fitness and was participating in circuit and strength training. However, his favorite physical activity, without a doubt, would have to be snowboarding.

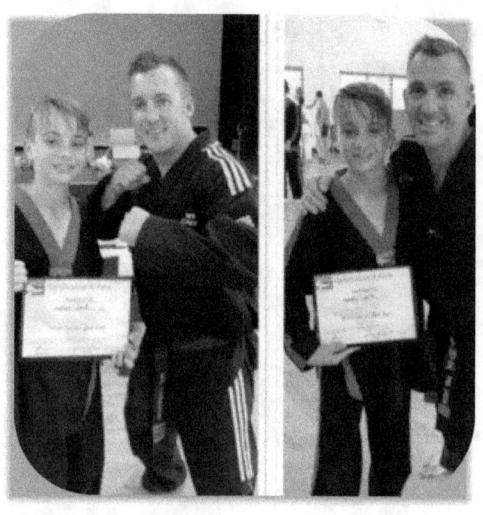

Aside from his weekly sporting activities Hunter's other passion is music. He loves to sing and play the guitar. He is a member of a wonderful music school and also the local Youth Theatre School of Excellence.

It is pretty safe to assume that Hunter had a full, rewarding, and sometimes hectic teenage boy's schedule. He has a wonderful sense of humor and there was always laughter in our home and something to look forward to.

As a baby, Hunter was born with severe bilateral talipes (club feet) and spent the first two years of his life, (from only eight hours old) in full length plaster casts on both legs. He received 4 major surgeries, the last of which was in 2014. Apart from a little stiffness and limited dorsiflexion in his right foot, he was perfectly fine, functioning like any other teenager and he could run extremely fast.

My husband Troy and I had made the decision to vaccinate our children as babies and again before they commenced school. To be honest, we had not really given the alternative much thought. Like most other parents we followed the rest of our fellow sheep and agreed to what we now understand to be called herd immunity.

I have always been very health conscious though and believed there was such a thing as over-vaccinating. As parents, we chose only the vaccines we deemed absolutely necessary. I have since discovered that our children are 'selectively vaccinated', a reference that once made me feel like a criminal. We said no to the chickenpox vaccine. All kids get chickenpox, it's like a rite of passage. We said no to the flu and meningitis vaccinations. I think there may be one other that was offered at school that we passed on.

Ironically, we had already refused the HPV vaccine for Hunter's sisters when the consent notes were sent home from school scheduling their vaccinations. Call it mother's instinct, but I had an awful feeling in my stomach and a very loud voice in my head about this vaccine. It had not been around long enough and quite simply, I did not trust it.

There had already been reports of adverse reactions in young girls in the United States, and whilst I did not look too deeply into these cases of Gardasil injury at the time, I knew enough to reject it for our daughters. I recall thinking even then, give it 20 years and there will be a huge increase in cervical cancer and infertility because of this vaccine. I was oblivious to the other possible forms of damage and injury that could arise.

Then the letters of consent started to arrive from school for Hunter's HPV vaccination in 2015. We really didn't give it much thought as Hunter was going to be away from school having post-surgery treatment on his right foot. Reminder letters and catch-up letters continued to arrive but we actually did not act on them at the time and Hunter did not receive the HPV vaccine.

In 2017 I was at our new GP with Hunter. She brought up the subject of the HPV vaccine and I told her that his sisters did not have it because I felt it was not safe and that he would not be getting it either. I mentioned that I had heard of many cases of young girls becoming seriously ill after receiving Gardasil in the United States.

Her response was, "It is a perfectly safe vaccine. The actual batches of Gardasil used in Australia are much better than the ones used in the USA. Ours has been developed more carefully."

Thinking about her statement now, I realize just how ridiculous it was.

But, all of this came at a time when we were not thinking clearly. Our lives had been turned upside down by a major injury to our daughter, and I had suddenly stopped listening to my inner voice, and my mother's intuition. My thoughts were consumed by other issues.

After much coercion, confusion and a lapse in concentration, we agreed to allow our GP to give Hunter the Gardasil vaccine. He received the first injection on the 11th of December 2017. He seemed fine and we didn't notice any specific changes or reactions. He had just started our summer holidays, so life was pretty relaxed.

I do remember thinking that he was more tired than usual, but as any parent would, assumed it was just part of being a growing, teenage boy. Nothing too unusual.

There was confusion at the time of his second dose regarding which type of Gardasil Hunter should receive and how many doses, given that Gardasil 9 had just replaced the original Gardasil and also Hunter was now 15 years old. There had been an appointment mix up, and we missed the rescheduled appointment also. Looking back now, all the warning signs were there, we had just been too preoccupied to heed them.

Hunter received the second and final dose of Gardasil 9 on the 22nd of June 2018. When the nurse was about to give him the injection, I had this overwhelmingly loud voice in my head, which very clearly said, "Do not do this!"

Not listening to that voice is my biggest regret. Apart from some minor soreness around the injection site on his arm, Hunter seemed fine. He had a small headache that evening, but nothing too alarming.

Tuesday July 17th was the athletics carnival at school. Hunter had an exceptionally great day and was very happy to have made the finals for his sprints and had won the 100 meter final, running 13 seconds. When I picked him up from school at 3.15pm, he was in excellent spirits and feeling quite chuffed with his achievements. He was looking forward to his session at Core-Strength Fitness that afternoon.

Within 5 minutes of getting into the car, he developed a painful headache, his vision was blurry and his right hand was numb. I decided it was probably best, after a long day of running, to skip the gym, and we headed home. Over the next 15 minutes, Hunter lost the feeling in his right arm and right leg. His headache was increasing in intensity and I noticed his speech had slowed a little. Not long after that, his upper back was burning and he had lost the feeling in his buttocks and left leg.

I was fearful that he was having a stroke and rushed him to our closest hospital. He was wheeled away immediately and a CT scan and MRI were done to rule out a brain bleed or blockage. Both tests were clear, but his symptoms were continuing to get worse. He was in excruciating pain and vomiting.

The doctor in charge believed Hunter had suffered a dehydration migraine and that the paralysis, headache, back pain and nausea were residual symptoms of the migraine, which would right themselves with time. He was kept in the hospital for overnight observation and given a saline drip and pain relief medication.

During the night, Hunter's pain increased and the paralysis worsened. He also became incontinent. He was very scared.

One of the nurses on duty came into his room at about 2am and

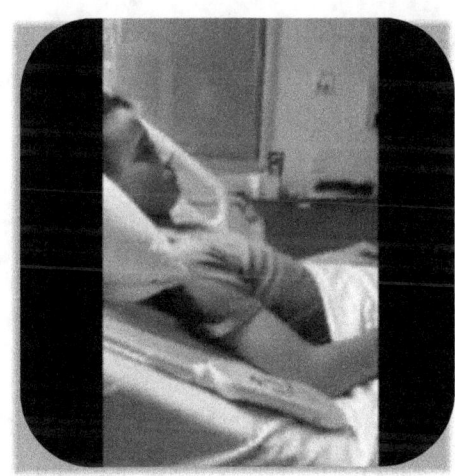

started questioning him about school, exams, friends, and bullies and asked him directly why he didn't want to go to school.

I was furious! This was not the right avenue to be exploring at this time, especially since no other tests had been carried out. I would have thought that only when all other possibilities had been exhausted, and only then, would these questions be asked.

This nurse did not know our son and that faking illness to skip out on school had never been on Hunter's radar. The nurse had no idea we were due to go snowboarding in New Zealand the following week, so the hospital was the last place on earth Hunter wanted to be.

The following morning Hunter was basically paralyzed from the waist down and in his right arm. He was not improving at all. The doctor decided to transfer him via ambulance to the University hospital. He arrived there late on Wednesday afternoon.

We were met by a young registrar who was the doctor on duty in the children's ward that evening. He agreed that Hunter had suffered a dehydration migraine but like the nurse at the previous hospital also strongly suggested it was psychosomatic. Since Hunter's paralysis was at both upper and lower levels of his body, he did not find his case a believable one. He did not carry out further testing. We had no answers.

Both my husband and I were baffled that they were not running any more tests, particularly as Hunter appeared to be getting worse. He was panicked and scared.

This was a kid who was not a stranger to hospitals or extreme pain because of his history with talipes, but he was writhing in pain right before our eyes. Late that night I looked at Hunter's spine and it looked like a question mark. It was extremely crooked and appeared to be in a massive spasm. I wondered whether he could have a slipped disc or a pinched nerve.

We called the doctor back and pointed out the severe irregularity in Hunter's spine. I asked for an MRI or X-Ray of his spine. He basically dismissed us and left Hunter with additional pain killers.

By Thursday morning the situation was still the same. Hunter now had pins and needles in his feet, he described this as a painful burning and buzzing just under the skin and he could not tolerate anyone touching him. The registrar and another new doctor were doing rounds that morning.

We were continually told what Hunter 'didn't' have, but no one was telling us what he 'did' have.

No more tests, X-Rays or MRIs had been carried out and his condition had been ruled as psychosomatic. We were beside ourselves and by mid-morning I told my husband to demand an MRI, even if we had to pay for it.

The registrar became annoyed, telling us we wouldn't find anything, but put Hunter on the hospital MRI list to shut us up. As his MRI had not been placed in the urgent category, Hunter was bumped down the list several times before finally having it done on the Friday, around mid-morning.

Not surprisingly, the results of the MRI were delivered by another new doctor. The Registrar had gone into hiding.

It turned out that Hunter had acute transverse myelitis and needed treatment urgently. He had several hyper-intense lesions in his spinal cord at T2 which extended from C5 to T1. This explained the paralysis in both his arm and legs.

At that point, the doctors were liaising with specialists from the Lady Cilento Children's Hospital in Brisbane regarding the best treatment options. High doses of intravenous steroids (methylprednisolone) were administered for three days.

At this time, it was also suggested he might have ADEM but it was less likely than ATM and a lumbar puncture was also done to look at his spinal fluid.

Hunter spent 9 days in hospital and during this time worked with a physiotherapist each morning. He slowly learned to sit up, stand and shuffle with the use of a full-length walking frame. He is a very determined young man and (although devastated that he needed to learn to walk yet again), by the time he left the hospital, was using crutches, albeit very slowly. He was making very small improvements each day, but they were improvements nonetheless.

One of the most difficult and frustrating things for Hunter to accept at this time was being unable to play the guitar. This is his passion and he went through quite a lot of emotions; heartbreak, depression, anger because he simply could not get his fingers to work. As you can imagine, there was a great deal of time to just sit and think whilst Hunter was sleeping in hospital.

It occurred to me then that it had only been three weeks since Hunter had received the Gardasil 9 vaccine and that was the only thing that had changed in his life and the only thing that could possibly be linked to his current situation. It was then that I googled Acute Transverse Myelitis and the Gardasil vaccine. The story of Colton Berrett appeared immediately.

From there I found links to literally hundreds of cases and stories of teens killed or injured by the HPV vaccine. I felt sick to my stomach, angered and completely grief stricken!

I read for days and days and researched everything I could. The more cases I read about and the more documentaries I watched on YouTube the more informed I became and the angrier I became. I spoke to Hunter's newest hospital doctor and suggested that Hunter's sudden onset of ATM was an adverse reaction to the Gardasil 9 vaccine. He agreed that it was more than likely.

He also told my husband that as a doctor he had to advocate for vaccines but he also believed I was right. Hunter's adverse reaction was reported to the national vaccine registry.

I then turned to Facebook on a whim and found three wonderful global support groups for devastated parents of Gardasil and vaccine-injured children.

I also spent many hours researching the best ways to help Hunter heal and how he could make a full recovery...if that was at all possible.

Hunter left the hospital on Day 9 and continued with oral steroids for about 2 months. During this crucial time, I realized pretty quickly that it was going to be entirely up to us to find ways to support the healing process. Unfortunately, GPs rarely acknowledge vaccine injury, let alone know how to help remedy the damage.

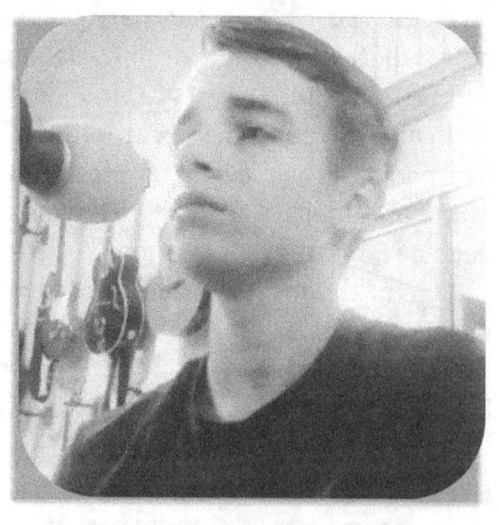

Most of them, I have since discovered, have not even read the package insert for Merck's Gardasil. They have no idea of the ingredients in the vaccine or the extensive array of adverse reactions, diseases and complications that can result from Gardasil, and that they are actually listed on the insert. I find it funny, and I am not laughing when I say this, that death is casually listed between chills and fatigue.

I have a good friend who sent me various links to information on natural ways to heal from vaccine damage. Within a week of being released from hospital Hunter's diet was completely organic, gluten-free, dairy-free, soy-free, sugar-free and for the most part grain-free. He is taking a myriad of natural supplements and vitamins to replace what has been leeched from his body; high-dose Ultra Vitamin C, Zinc, Magnesium, Liposomal D3, Iodine, Iron, Selenium, Probiotics, COD Liver oil, St Mary's Thistle, Diatomaceous Earth, Chlorella, Vital Greens, MCT oil, and various others.

Some days he really struggles with this strict dietary regime, but he understands the benefits to his recovery and that when it comes arguing with us, the subject is not up for debate.... ha, ha, ha!!

Hunter is having regular chiropractic adjustments, physiotherapy, and micro-current therapy. He has also had a session in a hyperbaric chamber and will be having more sessions over the summer holidays. He is on Metallothionein Promotion Therapy and recently commenced CEASE Therapy with an excellent Homeopath.

During his visit with the homeopath he was given an Oligo scan to determine the levels of heavy metals in his body. He has had a small regression since starting the CEASE Therapy but we have been assured that he will feel much better in the long term. It will just take some time and patience.

He had several weeks of a modified timetable at school and was attending half days for about 6 weeks.

It is still very early in Hunter's recovery journey and as I write this, he is only 4 months post injury. We are hoping and praying for a full recovery, but like most parents of Gardasil injured kids, we are constantly worried about what sinister health issue is lurking quietly beneath the surface, just waiting to rear its ugly head.

Prior to the slight regression we have seen since commencing Cease Therapy, he was regaining strength and energy. He is able to play the guitar again and sing. He recently performed in a tribute show of The Greatest Showman, in the role of PT Barnum for one of the songs. He was dancing a little, although still unsteady on his feet at times, but it was truly such a wonderful accomplishment for him and we were all so proud.

Hunter's biggest issue is fatigue. He gets tired a great deal and is constantly falling asleep in the car to and from school. He often has a long sleep after school and at times finds it difficult to find the motivation to complete various tasks. Some days are really good and other days are just awful.

On the down days he suffers from depression and anger at his situation, but we are all trying to stay as positive as possible and to just keep moving forward towards a full recovery. If we fill the house with laughter, silliness, happy times, and with various things to look forward to, it takes the focus off his illness and the negativity surrounding what has happened to him.

My husband is very pragmatic and his attitude has always been a 'we will just fix it' mentality. My research on how to do this and how to help Hunter heal continues.

The parental support groups I have joined have been a godsend and whilst I have never been one to advocate for the advantages of technology, I can definitely say, it has helped us to heal our boy. There are so many wonderful websites with information on healing vaccine injury and so many ways to connect with therapists, alternative-medicine professionals, and other parents. Hunter's healing journey could have been a very different story and perhaps not a very happy one, if it hadn't been for such incredible resources.

Thank you to the global communities of amazing people who have dedicated their lives to acknowledging vaccine injury, helping the healing process and for continuing to inform all of us on the risks of vaccines. I know we could not have done it on our own.

Whilst Hunter continues to improve at this point, there are no guarantees. We are just hoping for the best and will continue to fight for his health.

Like every parent in our situation, we worry every minute of every day and feel guilty every minute of every day. We are trying to redirect that anger, grief and energy into celebrating the positive milestones in his recovery and informing as many people as we can about the serious risks that accompany the Gardasil vaccine.

My hope is that other young men and women who have suffered and continue to suffer from Gardasil injury, and the parents who have lost their precious children or are coping with children who are seriously ill on a daily basis, find ways to heal physically and emotionally. I hope they find the strength to continue fighting, for themselves and for others. We have been violated beyond belief and we will never give up.

New Zealand

The New Zealand Ministry of Health's Immunization Technical Working group advised including HPV vaccines to the country's immunization schedule in November 2006. Before deciding on what age group to offer the vaccine to and how to structure the immunization program, the Ministry of Health looked at what was happening overseas and considered New Zealand's epidemiology. They also consulted public health experts and commissioned a survey to determine parental attitudes in their country.

In May of 2008 they announced their decision. Gardasil would be offered via a school-based immunization program as well as through primary health providers. For females ages 12-20 the vaccine would be paid for by the government. Those who were older would be offered the vaccine, but at their own expense.

1 September 2008, the vaccination program was launched in schools for those who had been born in either 1990 or 1991. Females of other ages could receive Gardasil at no cost through private health care providers until their 20th birthday.[107]

By September of 2009, there were three reports of young girls who had died mysteriously in their sleep shortly after Gardasil injections in New Zealand.[108] The health authorities said the deaths were not linked to the recent vaccinations, but the parents were not so sure. Thus, the controversy began.

By 2011, the school-based immunization was offered to girls between 12 and 13 years of age. Notices were sent to parents saying there would be a meeting with the public health nurse about HPV vaccines. Apparently, only the children were invited. Parents were

---

[107] New Zealand Ministry of Health; updated 23 Jan 2019; accessed March 2019

[108] Renata, R.; Gone After Gardasil: Jasmine-New Zealand; SaneVax.org; 14 Aug 2011

asked to sign and return a letter if they did not want their child to attend. At least one New Zealand parent was quite concerned about this meeting. She believed parents should have been asked to sign the letter if their daughter had permission to attend. In other words, she believed they should have been able to opt-in, instead of having to opt-out. She was also concerned that some girls might forget to talk to their parents about the meeting. If the children forgot, they would attend the meeting without their parents' consent or knowledge. She did not believe this was an acceptable practice.

Her statement to the local press was, "It is a decision that should be made by adults, not 12-year-old girls. At the very least parents should have been invited to attend the meeting to hear what information is being given to their children."[109]

In response to her frustration at not being allowed to make an informed choice regarding the medical intervention being offered to her daughter, she launched a website to provide parents with the information which was not being provided by the health authorities. She was determined to provide parents with enough information about the potential risks associated with HPV vaccines to enable them to make an informed choice.[110]

In July 2011, South Canterbury District Health Board chief executive Chris Fleming expressed concern about the low uptake of Gardasil saying, "I am very concerned that we have the lowest coverage for girls aged 12 and 13, and the district health board will be doing everything it can to ensure this improves. I also note that vaccination rates for older teenage girls in South Canterbury are much higher and in line with the rest of the country."[111]

September 2011, PSGR issued a press release calling on the Ministry of Health to "...immediately recall and review the potentially life-threatening Gardasil vaccine after 100% of 13 samples from several countries, including New Zealand tested positive for HPV DNA and may remain in circulation."

---

[109] Cogle, Fleur; Parents 'in cold' on vaccine meeting; Timaru Herald; 9 March 2011; accessed March 2019

[110] Lewis, Wendi; New Zealand Mom Launches Website Warning of Gardasil Dangers; Righting Injustice; 29 March 2011; accessed March 2019

[111] Bailey, Emma; Concern over low vaccine uptake; Timaru Herald NZ; 8 July 2011; accessed March 2019

The press release went on to state, "The discovery that some batches contain HPV DNA contradicts the Medsafe data sheets statement that the vaccine does not contain viral DNA: "virus-like particles are adsorbed onto an aluminium-containing adjuvant (amorphous aluminium hydroxyphosphate sulfate, or AAHS). Because the virus-like particles contain no viral DNA, they cannot infect cells or reproduce."

PSGR is a not-for-profit, non-aligned charitable trust composed of science and medical professionals.[112] Apparently, their plea was ignored. The HPV vaccination program continued uninterrupted.

An article in New Zealand's *Best Practice Journal,* published in April 2012 expressed concern over the fact that Gardasil uptake was lower than expected in the school-based vaccination program. The article suggested primary health care providers should offer information, address fears and concerns and promote uptake of HPV vaccines.[113]

In 2012, a coroner's inquest was held to examine the facts surrounding the unexplained death of an 18-year-old New Zealand girl. Testimony provided by Dr. Sin Hang Lee via an international video link before Coroner Ian Smith in Wellington NZ revealed the discovery of Gardasil HPV DNA fragments in post-mortem samples. Dr. Lee testified:

> *"The finding of these foreign DNA fragments in the post-mortem samples six months after vaccination indicates that some of the residual DNA fragments from the viral gene or plasmid injected with Gardasil® may have been protected from degradation in the form of DNA-aluminum complexes in the macrophages; or via integration into the human genome.*
>
> *Un-degraded viral and plasmid DNA fragments are known to activate macrophages, causing them to release tumor necrosis factor, a myocardial depressant which can induce lethal shock in animals and humans."[114]*

---

[112] PSGR press release; Recall and Review of Gardasil Vaccine; Scoop health; 14 Sept 2011; accessed March 2019

[113] Dr. Nikki Turner, Associate Professor Lance Jennings; The HPV vaccination programme: addressing low uptake; Best Practice Journal; BPJ: 43; April 2012; accessed March 2019

[114] Erickson, N; Breaking News: Gardasil HPV DNA discovered in post-mortem samples; SaneVax Inc.; 8 Aug 2012

Some journalists in New Zealand were paying attention to the controversy surrounding Gardasil and were willing to report accurately. In February 2013, the *Timaru Herald* reported that girls who had received Gardasil were sixteen times more likely to have a serious adverse reaction to it than they were likely to develop terminal cervical cancer. They reported that this raised doubts with critics about the value of this increasingly controversial vaccine. The *Timaru Herald* had submitted an Official Information Act (OIA) request which revealed that the death rate for cervical cancer in New Zealand between 2002 and 2005 was 1.95/100,000. This compared with 31 serious (life-threatening) adverse reactions for the 90,000 New Zealand girls who had received Gardasil vaccinations to date.

According to the article, the reactions being investigated included the death of an 18-year-old girl as well as reports of Bell's palsy and collapses.[115]

In April 2015, *Women's Day Magazine* in New Zealand had the courage to publish the story of a survivor of mysterious new medical conditions a young New Zealand girl experienced after the administration of Gardasil.[116]

On 1 January 2017, HPV immunizations became free for everyone, male and female, ages 9 to 26, including non-residents under the age of 18. Gardasil 9 is now the HPV vaccine of choice.[117]

According to the New Zealand Ministry of Health, between 2008 and January 2019, 300,000 New Zealander's have been immunized against HPV.[118]

How many of them had the opportunity to make an informed choice before being vaccinated?

How many of them have experienced new medical conditions after being vaccinated with Gardasil?

How many of them did not survive?

---

[115] Bailey, Emma; Opinions on Gardasil Clash; Timaru Herald; 24 Feb 2013; accessed March 2019

[116] Rapley, Kristina; Mum's heartbreak: What's happened to my girl?; Women's Day Magazine; April 2015; available on SaneVax

[117] Ibid ref #106

[118] Ibid ref #106

Adverse Events: Coincidence or Consequence?

By Krystal's mum, Ngatea, New Zealand

At 16-years-old, my daughter Krystal was a vibrant, energetic, sporty, positive young woman. Very strong willed and determined in

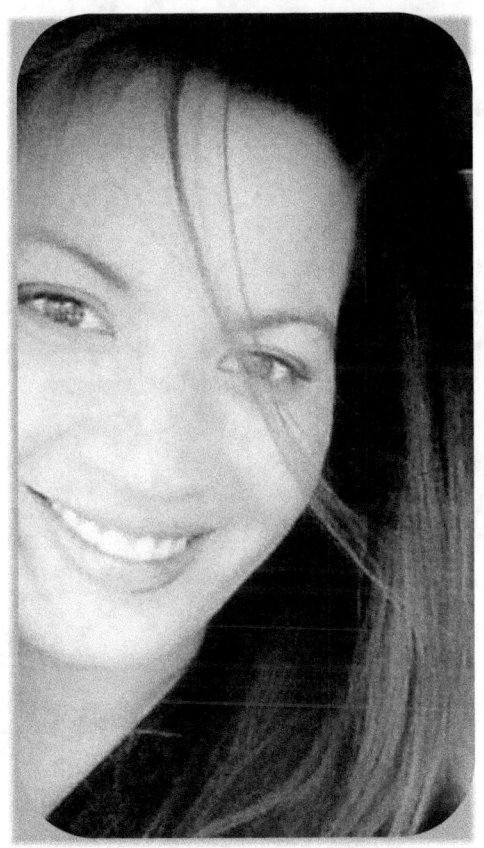

everything she set her mind to. Competed in the Weet-Bix Triathlon in 2005. She had played rep Netball for the previous six years as well as her Saturday team. She was actively involved in basketball, Touch, swimming and generally any sport available for her to participate in. One afternoon after I picked her up from school I remember her saying, "Thank you Mum, for having me." We were all happy and looking forward to a bright future. This was during the early winter of 2009.

On October 2, 2010, I made my daughter sit down and watch 'Close Up'[119] with me because they were showing a segment on Gardasil. I wanted her to watch the program because Krystal told me she had received two injections of Gardasil in the fall of 2009 without my consent. Since she was 16 at the time, she did not need my permission to receive the vaccine, but I wanted her to understand how important it was to make

---

[119] https://www.youtube.com/watch?time_continue=36&v=gM117iPkUjc

informed decisions. I had no idea that it was actually me who would become educated.

You see, Krystal's health had begun to deteriorate rapidly in November of 2009. We had no idea why. Although she had minor new medical conditions before November, they weren't like anything we were about to experience.

Soon her new symptoms included extremely severe migraines, muscle aches and pains, cold sweats, temperatures, nausea, lack of appetite, extreme fatigue and extreme moods. She could not think clearly and did some bizarre things which were totally out of character for her. She complained once of tingling in her hands.

She became very hostile and totally unreasonable to deal with. I even mentioned to friends and family that I would gladly have a houseful of teenagers any day rather than deal with what I had in my home at the moment.

If Krystal wasn't sleeping off an aggressive migraine, she was sleeping because she was so exhausted.

Her lack of attendance at school had me to the point where I didn't ring the school anymore to inform them. Consequently, she did not sit her two exams in December.

I honestly thought she was going through a 'teenage-itis' period, only this was an extreme one. Prior to becoming unwell Krystal had suffered from migraines but they were manageable, the new ones were not. I use the word extreme as everything she suffered from now completely knocked her flat.

Several times I checked in on her when she was sleeping just to make sure she was still alive.

Around Christmas 2009, Krystal had asked if she could find some 'Happy Pills' and I agreed to this as she was showing all the signs of severe depression and I was at a loss as to how to help her. Krystal was prescribed Citalopram hydrobromide tablets 20mg by her doctor on the 8 Jan 2010. She took 3 per day for approximately two weeks, then stopped as she couldn't tolerate them anymore. I tried to convince her to only take one each day, but was ignored. I tried to get her to see someone to talk about whatever was bothering her, but she refused.

Krystal had a Rep Netball Camp mid-January to attend but could not go. By this time, I thought there were little signs she was slowly recovering but she was still too unwell to participate.

Suddenly, after watching *Close Up*, I realized everything fit together. The dates the injections were given matched up with her health decline and her refusal to speak to someone because there was 'nothing' wrong. By nothing, I mean no situation that might cause her to become depressed, only a reaction to the vaccination triggering a downward spiral of her health.

As we had no idea she could be suffering an adverse reaction, we assumed there were situations in Krystal's life she was unable to control or, as the doctors put it 'unresolved issues'. Looking back, I believe the medical profession did not want to make a connection between HPV vaccines and serious health problems. It was far easier to put it down to unresolved issues causing depression in an otherwise fit and healthy young lady. They don't seem to see, or want to admit, vaccination may be a trigger in distorting thoughts as well.

It scares me to think what might have happened had we not seen this programme and I thank Rhonda and Stevie for speaking up and making us aware. My heart and prayers go out to them. Krystal was due for her third injection so I made the nurse put an alert on the computer that under no circumstances was Krystal to receive this shot. Krystal may have been another statistic. I believe Rhonda and Stevie saved Krystal's life.

We weren't ready to tell the full story when I sent the information above to Julie Smith, founder of "Off the Radar," 8 years ago. We knew there would be heartless comments and judgement. We were already hearing statements like: "Your daughters not sick;" and "You don't know what you're talking about." We could only imagine how bad it could become if our story became public. We were also scared of possible serious repercussions if our story were public knowledge. We decided it would be best for the family to concentrate our efforts on helping our daughter get well.

Sadly, Julie passed away in 2013 during her relentless efforts to help so many of us trying to find our feet post-Gardasil. She was a beautiful lady and is dearly missed.

Krystal is now 25 years old and has emerged emotionally and physically scarred but stronger in her quest to live, she continues to succeed daily.

We are now strong enough to be able to tell our story as a warning to others. We sincerely hope doing so will prevent others from following in our footsteps.

This is how it all began

During the winter of 2009, Mat was managing a 2800 cow farm between Taupo and Rotorua with up to 15 staff. I was supervising feeding calves then relief milking. Krystal was employed as a casual relief milker, with tractor work outside school hours.

Mat and I were working seriously long hours then coming home to Krystal's verbal abuse and aggression. We didn't know what was going on nor why. She seemed possessed. I couldn't tolerate Krystal's behavior anymore. To make matters worse, her younger sister, Ashley, followed suit. They are not only close in age but have a very special sisterly bond so Ashley thought Krystal's behavior was the norm and how she too should behave. I just wanted the noise to stop and no one was listening. I did the unthinkable as a mother and walked out on my family. 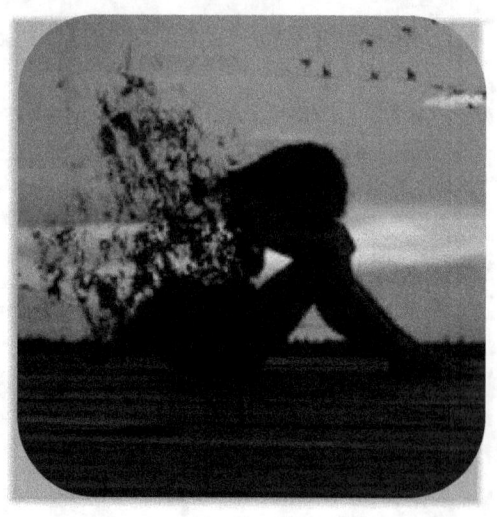 I returned after 8 days and we focused on Krystal. She was a very sick young lady.

Somewhere in between all of this, Krystal commented on how sore her arm was. I asked why and then she told me she had had a vaccine at school. I was only able to give her half my attention as our house was very busy, people coming and going, work etc. It did not click that this information could be important. A period of time later, she said she had had two shots and then I started to listen.

There was a time earlier in 2009 that I recall Krystal and Ashley coming home from school and handing me some information requesting for Gardasil to be given. Somehow I had already heard about Gardasil and not to get it. It did not sit well with me. I stated to them both it was a definite no and that they were not to receive it. As far as I was concerned that was the end of the matter.

After watching *Close Up* and making the connection with Gardasil, I contacted the local MP about my concerns and was brushed under the carpet. I spoke to Krystal's doctor on the phone twice, but he was not interested in Gardasil. On the first call, he told me Krystal had teenage issues and that she and I had communication problems. On the second call he stated, "Are you still going on about that?"

We were left with a sick daughter to tend to and no one to help.

We remembered Krystal's sickly grey shiny pallor at her last ever rep netball team trial out, when she struggled to stay on court for 10 minutes.

We remembered the nurse who administered the vaccine at her school, telling Krystal she would die if she didn't get it.

Only our family seemed concerned about the depression, anxiety, self- harming, mood swings like she was possessed, and all of Krystal's other new medical problems. In the initial stages we found her roaming the streets of our local town, Taupo, at 2.30 in the morning. While I talked to her on the phone to make sure she was safe, her father drove the 30 minutes to pick her up. She didn't want to be here.

Another night under similar circumstances, we eventually located her not far from home and had to call one of her friends to come around and coax her back home. Again, she didn't want to be here.

Other times when she would disappear for hours she would go to her favorite rock on the hill to sit and think. We got used to this over time. It was a lot easier once we knew where she was likely to go.

On top of this, Krystal finally told me she was cutting and showed me her wrists. She had been grabbing anything sharp to cut her wrists to overtake the pain she was feeling. Krystal would cover the marks with bangles so we never knew this was happening over those 12 months until she told me.

I didn't know anything at all about cutting at the time. This caught me completely off guard. It's hard to describe the feelings I experienced - a combination of grief, sadness, anger, loss.........flooding over me all at once. I felt like such a failure as a mother.

I regret slapping her to this very day and wish I could take it all back. How had we failed her? Why didn't we see the signs? Why was Krystal cutting? What does it all mean? So many questions.

Krystal had a great circle of friends and when she felt that she could, she went out with them. I asked that they keep an eye on her which they did. She just wanted to be and feel normal. When we had visitors Krystal would appear to be ok as she didn't want to let anyone know she was sick. It would take every ounce of energy she had to do this and when our visitors left she would fall in a heap and sleep. Exhausted.

I cannot recall how, but I happened to contact a lovely lady and her husband from further north towards Auckland. I was guided to take Krystal to a doctor and homeopath in Auckland. We organized what turned out to be a 15-hour round trip from Taupo. This was when Krystal's recovery began. She started detoxing and eventually we began to see a good day appear out of 7 bad days. Given more time her good days started to be more frequent and we saw some light at the end of the tunnel.

I also made a report to CARM, New Zealand's adverse event reporting system.

The side effects caused by this vaccine can be mild. They can be severe. You can confuse them with maybe the onset of the flu or like we did initially, possibly teenage problems, rebellion.

By now Krystal's schooling was over. There were times I would push Krystal out to work as I too thought this was just something she would get over.

When she was having semi ok times she would move back next door and on my way to work I would call in just to make sure she was still alive. That's how my days started.

April 2011, one week before her 18th birthday, Krystal broke the news to us that she was pregnant. What were we now facing? I was scared. But, her pregnancy turned out to save her life. It pulled her out of the darkest time she had ever experienced. She came alive. She became normal again, eating, sleeping, working and most important, laughing and happy.

During her pregnancy, she worked very hard to stop all self-harm and has never attempted it again. The thought of anyone knowing and someone in a health department misunderstanding our situation haunted us. We faced the distinct possibility Krystal could have her soon to be born child taken from her. We shared Krystal's story with her midwife who was wonderful and listened and respected our wishes on how we wanted the birth. Delayed cord clamping, no Vitamin K and no vaccines.

Then on the 8th Nov 2011 we met the wee boy who saved his Mum. Izaiah. However, it wasn't long before post-natal depression showed up. The pressure of not being able to breast feed was frustrating as much as we had persistently asked the lactation consultant to help through the midwife. More tears. Our only solution to this was to express and bottle feed. The lactation consultant wasn't perturbed by this at all and because Izaiah was putting weight on she decided to go on holiday. At 3-months-old, Izaiah had to have a hernia operation in his groin at Waikatio Hospital.

By the time Izaiah reached 8-months-old in 2012, we all moved to Patoka in the Hawkes Bay as an opportunity to manage a large farm in receivership came up and we couldn't turn it down.

It was here, just after Izaiah turned one that his father walked out on them both, leaving Krystal grieving and again spiraling into depression.

I had befriended a wonderful lady who was our neighbor. Unbeknown to us, she would play a pivotal role in reaching out to Krystal and we remain dear friends to this day.

We had many ups and downs, far too many tears and times I sat beside Krystal in her bed during bouts of depression telling her it will get better, to hang in there and she will feel better. Myself having to go to bed not knowing if she trusted my words and had the strength in herself to see the night through. Would she still be with us the next morning? I spent hours online trying to find more answers and help.

Krystal had been approached by "NZ 60 minutes" to tell her story but unfortunately they pulled out. "60 minutes" approached her again a while later only to pull out again. She also did a phone interview along with other Gardasil injured girls, with a reporter to be published in a newspaper. That too never made it to print. Why?

WE were healing Krystal. Not the doctors.

Sadly, for us after two years in Patoka, the farm sold and we had to move on. We moved 5 hours north to Wellsford in 2014 where once again Mat was managing and the owners eventually employed Krystal as 2 IC. Krystal was getting back to full time work, being a mum and playing Saturday netball.

It was here that she met her new partner Eti.

Ashley, Krystal's younger sister, was paramount in making the days successful. I referred to her as our 4th wheel. Without her, all things were not possible. Izaiah affectionately has always called her "Arni". Ashley herself faced her own serious health issue during 2014 and with hard work, great attitude and sheer determination, eventually overcame it in 2016.

Krystal and Eti announced that they were expecting. We were all a lot more relaxed this time around. Everything was going ok.

However, the owners informed us that their daughter wanted to come back to the farm the following season to contract milk so we needed to find new employment. We found positions just north of Taupo in 2015. Krystal secured a farming position on a family Trust farm only 5 mins away. Mat was settling in to the managing position when an opportunity came up to manage a family Trust farm adjoining Krystal's farm. So Mat applied for it and was given the good news that his interview was successful. We moved again. This was a farm that Mat's father had helped set up and we had all intentions of staying there.

However, it was here due to circumstances around us and way beyond our control, we were pushed to the brink. There was a very real possibility that we could have lost our house. Everything we had worked so hard for.

During an event here, Krystal almost went into early labor through shock but thankfully baby held on several more weeks. We finally met little Amarni Rose on New Year's Eve 2015 with the midwife respecting our birthing wishes.

Krystal was rushed back to the hospital by ambulance with complications a mere 24-hours after being released. 48-hours after Amarni Rose was born, thankfully everything became fine and Krystal was able to return home the following day.

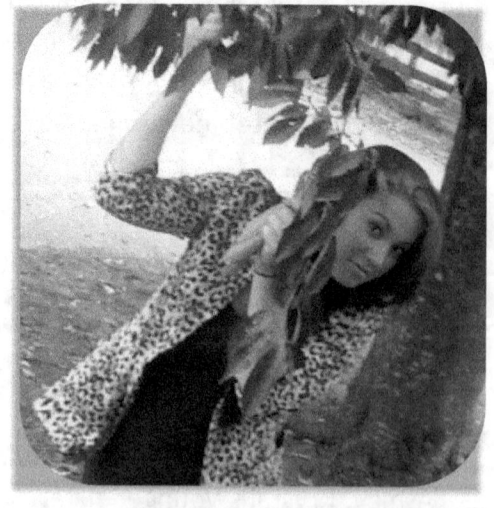

We were still immersed in dark days and stressful times with much more to come over the next two years but we did our best to make every situation better. Mat and I managed to secure a farming position in Millaa Millaa North Queensland, Australia and were due to fly out the first week of June 2016. It was a hard decision to make as we would be leaving behind the kids, not knowing how Krystal would cope. At the 11th hour a position came up in Okere Falls, Rotorua. This was another perfect opportunity for all of us and we turned the position down in Australia. Krystal was employed as Mat's 2 IC.

During October 2016 on the farm in Okere Falls Krystal became unwell. We just thought it was a bad flu as she had a sore throat with aches and pains so she took a week off work and obviously went to the doctor at A&E. She got a medical certificate and recuperated at home. The doctor took a throat swab which came back fine.

Over the following week she stated her left leg was swelling up from her knee. This was quite painful and she was having trouble moving around. Mat took her to A&E and she was sent home. They didn't know what it was. For the next 24-48hrs we watched the swelling travel up and down her leg and start to affect her right leg. By now we realized it was obviously fluid and moving very fast. Mat took her to A&E again. They treated her for a blood clot, sepsis arthritis and gout by draining her knee. Krystal called me from her hospital bed and I heard Mat yell in the background. He was watching the fluid move under her foot from her heel to her toes. It was rapid.

The pain was excruciating and with no answers from the doctors we immediately took her off for alternative treatment. Krystal was told she had Rheumatic Fever from undiagnosed Strep throat. I had to help her with the basics like toileting etc.... as she couldn't walk. Her father, partner, sister and I stepped in again to cover all areas of her life.

It turned out to be a very long road to recovery. From being immobile, to using crutches, to shuffling, to eventually walking without aid - with Izaiah teasing his Mum knowing full well she couldn't catch him. This made us all laugh.

Mat and I had tears in our eyes when we came home one morning from work to see her outside sweeping, unaided. Her crutches were leaning against the table.

During this time, I made a phone call to the A&E in order to try and speak with the doctor who failed to treat Krystal. I was not allowed to speak to him directly so asked the person on the other end of the phone to pass on a message. I wanted him to know that he had missed Strep throat and we were now treating her for Rheumatic Fever.

Several weeks later, Krystal received a referral in the mail to the Rheumatologist in Rotorua. I'm guessing the A&E doctor got my message and referred us. There had been no contact otherwise. At this appointment the specialist diagnosed Krystal with reactive arthritis and said to continue on with our treatment as obviously she was getting better and there was nothing else he could offer in the way of treatment. He also suggested we file an application for the mobile disability card so she could park close to shop entrances.

Krystal and Eti tell us they are expecting again. No surprises, this pregnancy went well also.

Once again we had to move as Mat's Managing contract was ending. This time we took on a Contract milking position in Coroglen, Whitianga. Krystal was taking time out on maternity leave so she and Eti along with Izaiah and Amarni Rose came to live with us. Eti found employment in Whtianga. Krystal was still having mobility issues.

Baby Eli was safely delivered 30th Aug 2017 in Thames Hospital by another midwife who was happy to respect our birthing wishes.

Eli has just celebrated his 1st birthday. We had intentions of employing Krystal on this farm but it was not viable. So once Krystal came to the end of her maternity leave, she and I found night time positions at the mussel factory in Whitianga. There were nights I had to help her because her knees made it difficult for her to do some of the tasks. Overall she coped well and enjoyed the comradery of the staff.

Unfortunately, working these hours created something I really wasn't prepared for. When we came home from our shift at 5:30am, Krystal would go to bed, I would milk with Mat then come home to watch the kids as Eti would take off to his work. I wouldn't get to 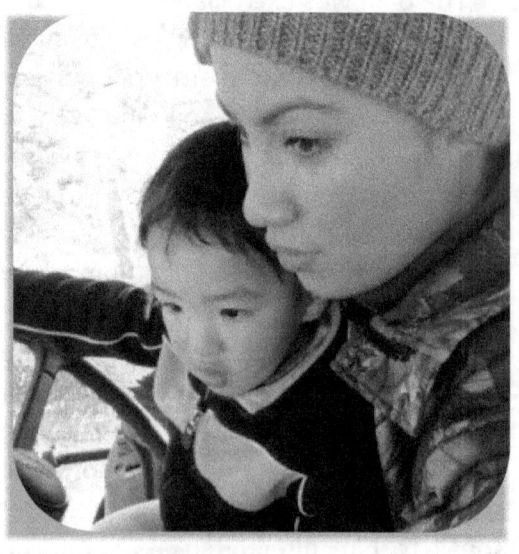 sleep until around 4pm. With only having approx. 5 hours of sleep per night I was now sleep walking.

We moved once again to a small town just out of Thames called Ngatea to a larger farm where Mat and I can remain self-employed, contract milking. This way, we can employ Krystal. This enables her to be independent, bring in an income and not be under the pressure of working for someone else who may not understand her situation. Work colleagues have commented on how 'lucky' Krystal is when she has extra days off. Little do they know. Thankfully no more night shifts.

Her partner relocated with us, initially forcing him to travel up to 2 hours to and from work. Then having to find work closer to home. Unfortunately, he has been made redundant twice in the past six months as there is very little construction work here in Ngatea/Thames.

Gardasil impacted us all.

No matter where our employment takes us, we always accommodate Krystal, Eti, and the children in order to make life work. We juggle and play tag on who babysits and who works.

It has taken a family team effort to enable Krystal to live as normal a life as possible. We don't know of any other way to get by other than how we are doing it. We also made the decision to sell our home six months ago to relieve some of the financial pressure.

Krystal and Eti, who is a builder, now have three beautiful children aged 1-year, 3-years and 7-years old. All unvaccinated.

Apart from Izaiah, the younger two do not have medical files. However, we believe Izaiah took the brunt of being first-born to a vaccine-injured mother. We have had to deal with only a couple of health issues he had where the medical profession has completely failed us again.

Over the past three years, Izaiah has suffered from a stomach problem causing high fevers and severe stomach pain but his stomach is soft. It caused him to be in bed for a week each time and seemed to occur monthly. He has had considerable time off school because of this. It's quite distressing for us all.

He was referred to a pediatric specialist in Thames. The specialist insisted Izaiah was constipated and that was all. This is after spending as little as five minutes with him.

Frustrated, Krystal and her partner returned to the doctors when Izaiah had another bout of this and the doctor simply supported the specialist. The recommendation was to continue giving him Paracetamol and keep him comfortable because he was simply constipated.

No. He was not constipated. We wanted answers. We wanted to know what it was. We will not be giving him paracetamol. By chance we discovered that Izaiah may have an intolerance to a certain spice or additive in food. So now we are careful with certain foods that he shouldn't eat. This is a work in progress for us, but I believe we are definitely on the right track. Since eliminating a certain food additive he has not had another episode.

Also, Izaiah has a stutter which came on suddenly prior to his stomach issue and we have had no help whatsoever from the medical profession in finding a cause. Panda's was mentioned to the specialist and once again ignored. Krystal and her partner were sent on their way.

We can only assume he suffered a traumatic situation at the childcare facility he was attending at the time which brought on this stutter as his speech was perfectly fine up until a particular day.

He has also had the measles, mumps, and chickenpox. Guess what............? Yes, he has survived!

These three children do not have pamol/paracetamol or antibiotics. They get sick occasionally but recover very quickly.

We are on constant watch to notice any signs of depression developing with Krystal. When they do, we act on it quickly. Whenever Krystal cannot walk, or can't use her arm, we cover for her on the farm. Whenever she is exhausted, we let her sleep and look after the kids.

Where do we go from here?

Our experiences over the last few years have truly opened our eyes. Surviving these circumstances has made us appreciate every day of life. This gratitude helps us cope with raising these three innocent children in a home of love and healing. It allows us to continue to face any new health issues Krystal may develop and learn to heal her.

We have been guided all the way through with Krystal and all four grandchildren. Yes, four. Ashley moved on last year to be with her partner. They now have a beautiful healthy son who is unvaccinated and about to celebrate his 1st birthday. He is going to be a big brother around July next year. For this, we will be forever grateful.

We were guided through hundreds of hours online, researching and connecting with other parents in similar situations. I honestly don't know what would have become of our family without the knowledge and connections we made during this time. Again, we are forever grateful for everything we learned and all of the wonderful people we met.

We don't know what the future holds for Krystal's entire health. We can only take one day at a time and do what we can each day.

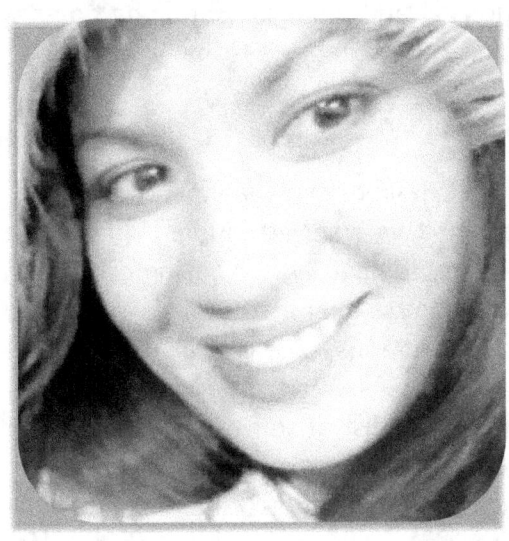 Krystal has had so much taken away from her. She grieves for the life that was but accepts her life as it is now. Of course, Krystal and her partner don't want to live with us. They want their own lives. They want a home where they can raise the children and not have to worry about whether Krystal will or won't be able to walk from day-to-day or be so exhausted she has to sleep.

We have been laughed and sniggered at when talking about what happened to Krystal. I have been trolled online because of our story. People we thought were friends ran the other way. To say Gardasil has taken a toll on us all is a gross understatement. Most of the medical profession has let us down tremendously. As soon as you mention Gardasil to a doctor they will not continue the conversation.

In October 2017, I asked IMAC (Immunization Advisory Committee) NZ on Facebook some questions and attached Dr. Lee's open letter including evidence of Helen Petousis-Harris trying to mislead Japan about the potential side-effects associated with HPV vaccines. Theo Brandt privately messaged me to inform me that I had offended his colleague and was now blocked from their site for asking inappropriate questions.

Hold on. Why would a private citizen be banned from a public information site simply for asking 'inappropriate' questions? If Helen could mislead Japan, what has she done to us in New Zealand?

What have we all been led to believe? What have we all been led to fear? Deceptive ploys? Follow the money!!

I shudder just thinking of what would have happened if Krystal had received the third shot of Gardasil. I firmly believe she would not be with us today had that been the case. We have had some very scary times during her recovery while facing the unknown. We survived stressful, exhausting, emotionally and financially draining times with a few dashes of laughter coming in-between.

This is how we live. This is our story.

Unless you experience a vaccine-injury you cannot judge.

I am not speaking out because we want attention. I speak out so no other family goes through what we have. After having come so far on our journey, the last thing we want to hear are people's opinions or the parroted rhetoric regarding vaccinations. The typical 'correlation is not causation' quote.

Before closing, I leave you with a list of some of Krystal's symptoms so you know what to look for should you suspect an HPV vaccine-injury. At various times, she experienced dizziness, memory loss, lack of concentration, brain fog, racing heart, joint pains, chronic fatigue, insomnia, headaches/migraines, nausea, vision problems, weight gain, bloating, irregular periods, heavy periods, extreme thirst and hunger, sweating and severe mood swings, and aggression. Her constant hunger is a concern. Upon waking she is starving which never ceases. She had cognitive issues, Bartonella infection, a sore arm at the injection site, chills, rashes, aches/pains, hair loss, Iron depletion, Reactive Arthritis, Epstein Barr Virus infection, and Encephalitis. Krystal has been showing signs of Lupus for quite some time, but a formal diagnosis has not been made. She is currently being tested for diabetes.

This is a list of the treatments which have helped Krystal: vitamin/mineral supplements, detox, color therapy, diet changes, homeopathy, and using essential oils.

As a parent, I can only suggest everyone to stop listening to the herd and start researching. Listen to families and ask questions. Spend time examining vaccine ingredients. Read the package inserts. We have all been playing Russian roulette with our children's lives. This is not acceptable.

Please, don't wait until something happens to your child. Become an informed medical consumer!

Footnote: Since writing our story, Eti is now working in Melbourne, Australia. Krystal has chosen to move over there also with the kids and make the most of this opportunity. Mat and I give them our full blessing in this major move. Gardasil has consumed so much of our lives. Life is so short and precious, given our experience, Krystal is as prepared as she can be. We don't want to focus on the negatives but if anything were to happen we are only a 3-hour plane trip away.

The Worst Decision of my Life

Submitted by Deborah Robson, Auckland New Zealand

Our previous life was one of a normal 12-year-old girl. Attending

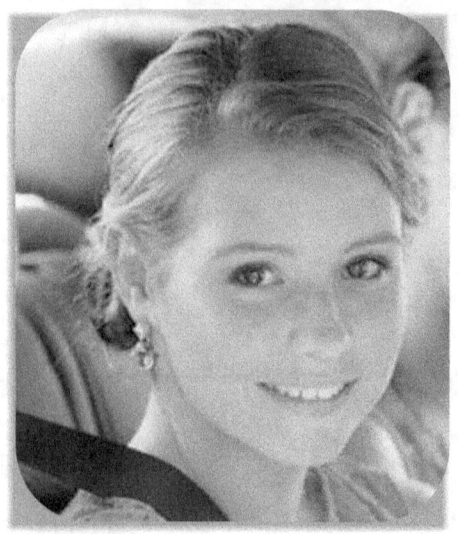

school, playing sports, learning the guitar, hanging out with friends, enjoying family get-togethers, looking forward to family outings, exploring new places, cultures and food, laughter and happiness.

All that was taken from us in 2014, when I made the worst decision of my entire adult life. I signed the consent form for my then 12-year-old daughter to have all three Gardasil vaccinations.

At the time, this decision was an absolute no-brainer for me, or so I thought. My daughter was fully vaccinated and had met all her milestones as a child. Ironically I had been diagnosed with cervical cancer in 2003 and had to have an emergency full hysterectomy leaving me unable to have any more children. My GP endorsed this vaccine for my daughter, especially given my circumstances. I didn't do any independent research. I relied on the experience and knowledge of my GP, because we were brought up to put our full trust in our doctors. They know what they are talking about right? This couldn't be further from the truth.

12 March 2014, my daughter received her first dose of Gardasil at school. There were no immediate symptoms, simply a bit of pain at the injection site and her shoulder which soon subsided.

28 March, my daughter had a severely infected throat. We consulted our GP and she was put on antibiotics. Come the 14th of April my daughter was admitted to our Children's Emergency Hospital with what they said was some kind of viral illness. She had myalgia (pain) in all

four limbs, fever, frontal headache, dizziness on sitting and standing, epigastric pain, and photophobia. She was discharged that evening and sent home. Her symptoms subsided, and we carried on with normal life.

21st May 2014, she was given the second dose of Gardasil at school. Again, no immediate reaction or obvious symptoms.

On the 25th June, we visited our GP as my daughter was suffering from shortness of breath on waking with a high fever, she was again admitted to hospital and discharged two days later with a diagnosis of pneumonia and a lower respiratory tract infection, along with severe abdominal pain.

Again after a few weeks, my daughter's symptoms subsided and we returned to our daily lives.

Never once did I consider these symptoms might be reactions to the vaccine as they were not immediate and usually a good month later. Little did I know that this is very common, symptoms can raise their ugly head months, even years later.

10th September 2014 was the third dose. This is the one that completely destroyed my daughter's life. None of our lives would ever be the same. The sheer horror and heartbreak that was about to blow our family apart was lurking just around the corner.

We again visited our GP on the 8th of September for another strange virus. This time we were not sent to hospital. Around this time, I also noticed my daughter becoming very reclusive. She didn't want to see her friends and didn't spend very much time at all out of her bedroom. She had become a completely different girl.

October the 19th was her 13th birthday, but she wasn't at all interested in celebrating which rang huge alarm bells. I visited her school to discuss this with her teachers and the school councillor. The reply I got was, "Yes, we have noticed she is not herself. She doesn't participate in class like she used to and has become very 'dark'."

So many thoughts were racing through my head: Was she being bullied? Are drugs involved? Surely not drugs, my daughter was not that type of child. She and I have such a close bond. All I could do was keep a close eye on her and try to talk to her, which was not an easy option.

1st October, another GP visit, this time my daughter was suffering from severe anxiety attacks, she could see and hear people no one else could and was extremely frightened. We then received a referral to see a child psychologist to help my daughter.

My daughter started to self-harm, cutting herself on her wrists. When I asked her about this she said, "Mum it relieves stress."

Of course, this was something I could not fathom in a million years. It would have never entered my head as a teenager to harm myself. Now she was aware I knew this was happening, she started cutting herself on the outside of her thighs, so it was hidden. That is until the day I walked into the bathroom as she was getting out of the shower. My heart sank, I felt hopeless and so frightened, I had absolutely no idea what was going on in my child's head or why.

31st October 2014, Halloween, trick or treat alright, this was the beginning of our nightmare. This was the beginning of hell. My daughter came to me an absolute shaking mess. Floods of tears and absolutely terrified. She said she could see and hear two people and said to me, "Mum, they are hurting me."

I can't even begin to explain what went through my head. Drugs? Was she seeing ghosts? What on earth was happening?

I asked her, "How are they hurting you?"

Her reply was, "They are hitting me. Look Mum!"

Sure enough, she had a big red welt on her right leg. I immediately put her in the car and took her straight to our GP. I had never ever seen my daughter in such a state. Actually, I had never seen anyone in a state of absolute terror and confusion like my daughter was that night.

She would not let me come into the meeting with our GP, so I sat outside by myself, not knowing what was happening to her. The meeting finished and our GP asked me to come in and have a talk with him. The nurse stayed with my daughter while I was with our GP.

He said to me, "She has had a psychological breakdown and we need to admit her to hospital. A Psych team will visit your house in the next few hours to evaluate the family and look at the best possible care for her prior to admission."

I was a complete mess. Why is this happening? How did this happen? I couldn't process this. Honestly, I felt like I was in a movie and this was all going to turn out to be a bad dream.

Two hours after we got home the Psych team arrived. We were all interviewed about our family life. I felt like this was an interrogation as we were interviewed in separate rooms. My God, we are not criminals; we do not abuse our child; we love her more than anything in this world. Please tell me what is going on. After the evaluation team came to the conclusion that we lived in a loving household, they admitted her to our children's hospital for evaluation.

We spent all night in the emergency department running tests, scans, and more interviews. 4.30 the next morning, my daughter was admitted to the children's psych ward.

With no sleep and a million things running through my brain, I just could not process this. I slept on the floor for a couple of hours until the day began in the ward and I could talk to doctors and psychologists. They really had no idea what was happening to my daughter.

The environment she was in was frightening. These children were from abusive families, families that didn't care for their children. Children who had been in and out of homes, and other facilities, children who had been beaten, children who had given up on life.

As the next week progressed, my daughter became more disorientated and frightened. She was so scared she was going to hurt someone because the voices kept telling her to hurt people. She wouldn't even let me see her as she was terrified she was going to hurt me. I would drive to the hospital every day and try and see my daughter.

On the second day I entered her room, she was sitting on her bed rocking in the corner. Her eyes were dark. I had never seen anything like it. It was as if some dark entity had taken over my daughter's body. As I approached her, she screamed at me to get back. 'Don't come near me! Leave her alone! Get out, get out!" she screamed at me.

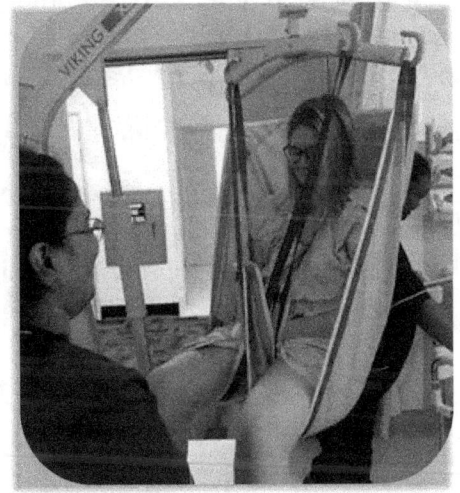

I had to go. I didn't want to leave her in that state. I was a mess. The nurses came to calm me down and said they would take care of her. She was put on I don't know how many psych medications and they told me they would check on her every hour.

The next day I drove to the hospital, parked my car and texted her to see if she would see me. "No Mum I don't want to see anyone."

I sat in my car all day hoping she would change her mind. Later that day she did. She wanted a cuddle and was crying. She told me the night before she had tried to strangle herself with her shoelaces. The voices kept telling her, "You are worthless and nobody wants you, kill yourself."

The feeling of despair is something I can't begin to explain. My girl had tried to take her own life and nobody had any idea what was going on. I didn't want to leave her there alone, she was only 13 years old. She needed her Mum. Again, I had to deal with the torment of leaving her and go home.

The next few days were much the same, I would drive to the hospital every day hoping she would want to see me. Each day I managed to see her for a short while. During one visit I learned she had poured a cup of boiling hot chocolate over her head because the voices had told her to. She could still feel these entities hurting her and would lash out at them to make them go away.

This was the worst week of my life, my daughter was in a psych ward wanting to kill herself, and I was an absolute wreck and still no idea why.

Five days after she had been admitted to the psych ward, I received a phone call from the hospital asking where I was and could my family and I please come in for an emergency meeting. My heart sank, is my daughter alive was my first response.

"Yes, she is fine. We want to talk to you about her tests."

It turned out that a number of specialists had a round-table meeting to discuss my daughter's case and had re-examined her MRI Brain scan. This showed swelling of the hippocampus area of her brain. They now realised the hallucinations and voices were a medical problem. They also said they had found a rare oligoclonal band in her blood tests and would transfer her to the neurology ward.

We were not prepared for the next two months. My daughter was admitted from the 31st October through to the 20th December that year.

More tests and scans were done. The new diagnosis was Limbic Encephalitis, oligoclonal bands present, auditory hallucinations with short-term memory loss. My daughter's short-term memory had become so bad that a nurse could walk in the room and introduce herself, two minutes later come back and my daughter would have absolutely no idea who she was. Her headaches were debilitating and she was still in a state of fear and wanting to kill herself. Because of this the hospital would move her back to the psych ward in between treatments as they did not have the staff on the neurological ward to cope with this type of behaviour.

I tried to tell the staff this was the worst place for her. She does not belong in a psych ward; she needs medical treatment. I offered to stay 24/7, but of course I couldn't possibly stay awake 24/7. I had to come to terms with the fact that this was how it had to be until they could work out what was going on and find a way to help her.

After numerous neurological investigations, my daughter was admitted to intensive care for Plasmapheresis and IVIG, she needed to have five treatments.

I was told this is the gold standard treatment and would take her immune system back to zero, back to a baby's immune system when it is born. This way hopefully we would be killing off all the bad cells and new healthy cells would be produced to re-boot her entire immune system.

A very large central line was put into the side of her neck to extract her blood into a machine which removed her plasma which was then replaced with new healthy plasma. Unfortunately, this gold standard process made no improvement.

December 20th 2014, my daughter had been discharged from hospital and was at home with our family. My partner came to me with an excruciating tooth ache and asked where the pain killers were, something he never takes, as he hardly ever gets sick. I said to him take some of Kate's Codeine they are in the pantry. He turned to me with an empty container in his hand.

I immediately flew into the lounge where all the kids were watching a movie. Kate was under a blanket with her eyes rolling to the back of her head hardly responsive. In a state of shear panic I called emergency and we had an Ambulance arrive very soon after.

I can't describe the fear I felt at this moment, my daughter had tried to take her own life. My poor girl who had recently turned 13 could not cope with this nightmare anymore. We were lucky. She pulled through this attempt on her life. She told me 'they told her to kill herself'.

December 24th Christmas Eve 2014 the hospital started chemotherapy, as a last resort.

Kate had a massive reaction and we had to pull the pin, the infusion was re-scheduled for the 29th of December. There were three or four more infusions, until we instructed the hospital to stop, this was making Kate very sick. In hindsight, we were loading her up with more toxins, something her body wasn't able to process.

Christmas that year was spent in and out of the hospital or at home bedridden with chronic headaches and trying to deal with auditory hallucinations constantly.

22nd March 2015, Kate tried to take her life once again. By this stage I had removed, or tried to remove, everything and anything in our home that could cause her harm and was sleeping constantly with one eye open.

There was only one bottle of codeine in the house, completely hidden. To this day I have no idea how she found that bottle. I was in the kitchen cooking and heard a blood chilling scream come from my daughter's room. I ran to her room to find her sobbing with an empty pill container in her hand saying, "I am sorry they made me do it. I tried to pick up my phone to call you but every time I did they hit the phone out of my hand."

Another frantic call to emergency, this time she had taken 60 tablets, this was serious. By the grace of God, she pulled through again. I am pleased to say this was the last time she attempted to take her life.

We endured months of constant ice-pick headaches, numerous

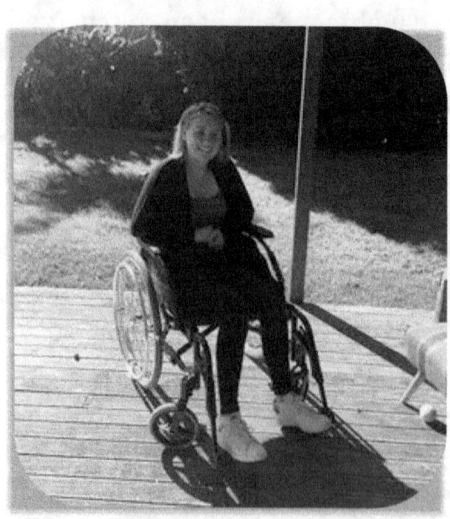

hospital admissions for acute abdominal pain, constant dry retching, Kate was unable to eat or drink for days at a time.

Then came the chronic period pains: diagnosis possible endometriosis. Because of her age they did not want to do an internal investigation. However, by early 2018 her pain had become so bad we went ahead and found endometriosis of the bowel, uterus and colon. Kate had surgery to remove this.

During the beginning of 2015, joint pain, chronic fatigue, limb weakness and tingling started to occur. These symptoms became a constant daily battle. Kate would collapse suddenly with no warning and be too weak to get back up. She could no longer attend school. She couldn't even walk to our letter box unaided.

Night terrors became regular, they were so frightening to Kate, that she would wake from the experience feeling what had happened was so real. It got to a stage where she was petrified to go to sleep. Once she was asleep, she was unable to stay asleep.

Anxiety and depression became much worse. I now had a daughter unable to attend school, losing her friends because really what 13-year-old child could understand what was going on with our daughter? Nobody knew, not even the medical professionals.

September 2015, Kate was again admitted to the children's hospital and diagnosed with Central Neural Sensitisation syndrome (Chronic Pain Syndrome). Their answer to this was let's dose her up on mega pain blockers and anti-depressants. After two weeks in hospital unable to walk, Kate was transferred to a home for disabled children where we spent the next three weeks 24/7. Every day was intensive therapies, Kate was absolutely exhausted and suffering in so much pain.

The remainder of that year was spent bedridden, in and out of a wheelchair, trying to function day by day.

My daughter's life had been taken from her and I as a Mother felt absolutely helpless. Any spare time I had was spent researching the adverse effects this vaccine has had on thousands of girls worldwide.

I joined a Facebook group of parents who were all experiencing the same destruction of their child's life after vaccinating with Gardasil. Many nights I sat and cried, reading story after story feeling so guilty, I had made this decision, with no research whatsoever. I had trusted in our medical system, something I will never do again.

2016 was much the same, multiple hospital admissions for chronic pain, blood pressure issues, headaches and joint pain.

In April of 2016, Kate and I decided we would take a weekend away and visit good friends which was an hour-and-a-half flight away. Just over half an hour into the flight Kate grabbed my leg, she was slumped in her seat, going blue around the mouth and unable to breathe properly. Thankfully there was an emergency doctor on board who took over and managed to get us safely to our destination where the ambulance was waiting to take us to the local hospital's emergency department. Not the way we were planning to start one of our only weekend away in a long time.

Again, test results came up with nothing. She was diagnosed with tachycardia and shortness of breath then discharged.

The following week, Kate was again admitted with chest pains and palpitations and referred to a cardiologist. Once again test results came up with nothing remarkable.

June 2016, Kate was admitted to hospital with chronic back and rib pain. Diagnosis: costochondritis 2nd and 3rd Rib /osteochondroma.

November 2106 Kate was admitted to hospital with Central Neural Hypertension, chronic headaches and hallucinations, she was discharged 10 days later.

Again, another Christmas spent, in constant pain, depressed, and wanting to give up.

My daughter was so lonely and heartbroken, she was broken. We all were.

2017 started much the same way as every other year since her Gardasil injections, hospital admissions for hip problems, and further admissions for chronic bilateral leg pain. Once again Kate was bound to a wheelchair unable to walk or move on her own, dealing with constant excruciating pain.

June 2017, Kate's high school ball was looming. She was still bound to a wheelchair and succumbed to the fact she would be attending in her wheelchair. This is when I found a fabulous centre called Neurophysics who worked with Kate on a holistic level. Within 2 weeks she was walking again. I am happy to say Kate did attend her school ball, no wheelchair in sight. All be it a hard night for her to get through, I am so happy she will have those memories forever.

July 2017 my world again came crashing down. Kate needed to have her appendix removed. Whilst under anaesthetic Kate had a massive anaphylactic reaction to the muscle reversal drug and stopped breathing. I received a phone call from the anaesthetist saying Kate had been rushed to intensive care. I was not able to see her for another two hours. That was probably the longest two hours of my life. I felt sick to my stomach walking down to Intensive Care. My daughter had been intubated, had a central line in her neck and IV lines all over her body. They kept her on life support for the next 24-hours.

Fast-forward to today, October 2018, are we out of the woods yet? No, we are not, and I don't honestly know if we will ever be.

My daughter's teenage years have been taken from her. Her health has been taken from her. She will never be the same child she was before Gardasil.

The one thing I do know is my daughter is a fighter. She is strong and has a beautiful heart. After everything she has been through, I know she will go on to do wonderful things in this world.

If you ask me, does the risk outweigh the benefit when it comes to Gardasil?

Absolutely NOT! I consider this vaccine dangerous and in some cases deadly. To consent to this vaccine is playing Russian roulette with your children's life.

This is something I have had to come to terms with. The terrible guilt has been unbearable at times. To watch your child in so much pain and feel so helpless, is something no parent should ever have to experience. These are our babies, they are so young with the rest of their lives ahead of them.

Please, protect your child's health. Do your research.

CHAPTER 5

Africa

South Africa

South Africa has a high cervical cancer rate with an incidence rate of 43.5/100,000 and a mortality rate of 19.1/100,000. Cervical cancer ranks as the 2nd most frequently diagnosed cancer among South African women.[120]

In 2000, South Africa launched a national screening program which offered three Papanicolaou smears per lifetime starting after the age of 30 with 10-year intervals between screens.[121] However, the screening program was offered on an opportunistic basis, meaning either the woman had to ask her healthcare provider for the test, or the healthcare provider had to suggest the test when she was in the clinic for other reasons. In stark contrast to an organized screening program with recall reminders and follow-up, opportunistic screening is not necessarily checked or monitored. It was probably no surprise when the South African screening program suffered from low uptake, thus limited success.

---

[120] South Africa: Human Papillomavirus and Related Cancers, Fact Sheet 2018; ICO/IARC; accessed March 2019

[121] Matthys H. Botha, Carine Dochez; Introducing human papillomavirus vaccines into the health system in South Africa; Vaccine Volume 30, Supplement 3; 17 Sept 2012; accessed March 2019

HPV vaccines, both Gardasil and Cervarix, were approved for use in South Africa in 2008. Since they were only available via private pay uptake was quite low. Government officials believed other factors contributing to the low uptake rate included public lack of knowledge regarding the link between HPV infections and the development of cervical cancer, as well as the fact the general population had no experience with vaccination programs targeting adolescents.

An editorial in the January 2015 edition of the *South African Medical Journal* proposed a possible solution to solving the low cervical cancer screening rate while introducing HPV vaccines into the national immunization program. Simply link the opportunistic screening of mothers/caregivers to the HPV vaccination program. The authors spoke of Vaccine and Cervical Cancer Screen (VACCS) pilot projects which experimented with just that option. They combined the vaccination of adolescent girls against HPV with cervical cancer screening interventions offered to their female caregivers.[122]

For the first VACCS demonstration project, 19 primary schools in low socioeconomic areas of the Western Cape and Guateng provinces were chosen to participate. School is compulsory in South Africa and virtually universal, so the project was almost certain to reach every girl eligible for HPV vaccination.

Basically, this is how the project was conducted: letters were sent home with all students in grades 4-7 asking for them and their parents to come to an HPV information evening. The first step was to obtain parental permission to attend. Once there, the parents were interviewed, then asked to sign permission for an educational session. At the end of this session, the parents and the children were asked to sign consent for HPV vaccinations. Although both were asked to sign, any child 12 years of age or older could legally sign the consent form without her parents' permission. At the same meeting, the mothers or caregivers were offered the opportunity to participate in a cervical cancer screening program.

If the parent did not sign the consent form at the meeting, they were sent home with an information packet containing an additional consent form in case they changed their mind at a later date. Parents

---

[122] Botha, MH, Richter, KL; Cervical cancer prevention in South Africa: HPV vaccination and screening both essential to achieve and maintain a reduction in incidence; SAMJ Volume 105; January 2015; accessed March 2019

who chose not to attend the information sessions were also sent another packet of information with a consent form they could sign if they chose.

Out of all the parents invited to participate, the consent rate was 59%. The rate of consent for the parents who attended the information events was much higher, at 87.5%. When all was said and done, 63.7% of the target population in the Guateng schools had been vaccinated as well as 53.9% of the targeted population in the Western Cape schools. The manufacturers of Gardasil and Cervarix had donated the vaccines needed to complete the project.[123]

The August 2014 edition of the *South African Medical Journal* published a letter to the editor submitted on behalf of no less than twenty members of the South African HPV Advisory Board singing the praises of HPV vaccines. One of the most prominent statements in this letter was, "A vaccine is only approved after extensive clinical trials prove that the benefits of vaccination outweigh any possible risks associated with it."

Evidently this team of HPV experts did not read the background papers which the HPV vaccine manufacturers submitted to the FDA prior to gaining marketing approval.

After a rather long explanation of how marvelous HPV vaccines are and how efficiently potential adverse reactions are tracked after vaccination, the article went on to issue a rather strange warning. The letter stated:

> *"It can be expected that anti-vaccine campaigners will take advantage of the HPV vaccine debate, focusing on concerns about safety and isolated reports of adverse events temporally related to vaccination. It is imperative that healthcare professionals are well informed so they are able to answer questions and dispel the myths surrounding HPV vaccination in order to ensure maximum vaccine coverage and herd immunity."*

---

[123] Botha, M., van der Merwe, F., Synman, L., Dreyer, G. (2014); The Vaccine and Cervical Cancer Screen (VACCS) project: Acceptance of human papillomavirus vaccination in a school-based programme in two provinces of South Africa; SAMJ 105(1). 40-43; doi:10.7196/SAMJ.8419; accessed March 2019

At the time, there appeared to be no debate surrounding HPV vaccinations in South Africa. Why did the authors feel compelled to issue such a warning?[124]

In April 2014, South Africa initiated a national public school-based program to provide free HPV vaccines to all Grade 4 girls over the age of 9. More than 16,000 public schools throughout South Africa with an eligible population of 408,273 young girls were targeted. Out of that cohort, 353,564 (86.6%) were given their first HPV vaccine injection. They would be scheduled for the second dose the following school year.

The interesting thing about this program was it included an assessment of media coverage. Beginning several days before the start of the campaign and for several days after its conclusion, virtually all media coverage from March 1 to April 30, over 900 print, broadcast, and online media sources was reviewed. This included 80 newspapers, 291 community publications, 95 magazines, 37 radio stations, and 13 television stations. A media analysis company was hired to assess the media coverage during the campaign and rate the communications as positive, neutral, or negative.

Ostensibly, this analysis was supposed to provide information that would help other countries nip 'rumors and fake news' in the bud. Their analysis was interesting though. They found that 38% of all media coverage was positive, 55% was neutral, and only 7% was negative. The second interesting piece of information was that 70% of all positive media coverage was in March, before the campaign started; while 59% of all negative media coverage was in April, after the campaign was underway.[125] Mainstream media attention primarily focused on vaccine safety which dominated social media. The claim was made that this focus had 'a strong global imprint, as much of its content was sourced from anti-vaccination lobby groups and influential "victim" support groups based outside of South Africa.'

The basic conclusion was preemptive strategies must be developed so this type of 'focus on safety' did not interfere with future HPV

---

[124] Letter to the editor of SAMJ; HPV vaccine: Can we afford to hesitate?; submitted on behalf of 20 members of the South African HPV Advisory Board; SAMJ Vol 104 No. 8; Aug 2014; accessed March 2019

[125] Delany-Moretlwe S, Kelley K, James S, et al. Human papillomavirus vaccine introduction in South Africa: implementation lessons from an evaluation of the national school-based vaccination campaign. Glob Health Sci Pract. 2018;6(3):425-438; accessed March 2019

vaccine uptake. One has to wonder why concerns over vaccine safety, regardless of the source, fail to take precedence over vaccine uptake. Shouldn't the top priority be public health and safety?

Evidently, at least one South African citizen thought so. She sent the following questions to the Cancer Association of South Africa (CANSA) on 9 August 2015:

> *"Could you please let me know why CANSA is supporting the use of the HPV vaccines when these are now proven to be deadly? Several hundred young women have died because of this vaccine and thousands more are permanently disabled or battling with chronic health problems. This vaccine has NEVER been proven to prevent cervical cancer. They are not just useless, they are dangerous – why is South Africa using them? And why does your web page not list the potential side effects?"*

My Personal Journey

By Shaina Wheeler, South Africa

I am Shaina Wheeler. Allow me to tell you a little bit about myself. I am an eighteen-year-old girl, in my final year of school. I have dark brown hair, blue eyes, and a curvy body (much to my dismay). These are all of the things that you see when you look at me. Everybody sees what you appear to be, but very few people see who you actually are.

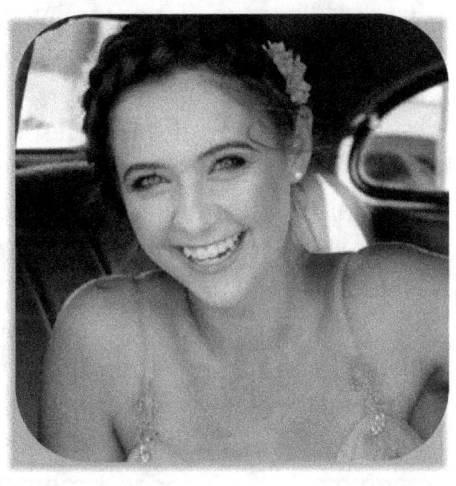

These things listed above are the things I appear to be, however I am slightly more multi-facetted than that. From the outside I am the girl mentioned above. I do a pretty good job at playing the 'I have my life together' character.

I recently attended a ceremony at my school, where individuals were being awarded for their achievements. During the ceremony I started to reflect on my last two years of high school and all of the moments leading up to this day - all of the tests, exams, sports games, camps and just normal days of school. I had the desolated thought of what my life could've been like, and how this day could have been so different for me. Let me explain.

I was once the girl who played all the sports, the girl who was a part of every single event or game that was available to me. I was always eager to do something new and exciting. Being an athlete ran in my blood. I was so competitive, continually wanting to improve myself, to be something faster, stronger and smarter. Looking back, that's probably why I loved sports as much as I did... I could never get bored, there was always room for improvement. I loved pushing myself and my body, to extents that seemed completely out of reach. I had an inconceivable passion for sports. However, this vehemence that was inside of me did not only come out on the sports field.

Some would say that I am a social butterfly - I don't think that there is anything I savor more than spending time with the people I love. It is in my nature to impress the people around me. I went through my school career trying to make everybody happy, even if it wasn't necessarily my responsibility. I never ever wanted anyone to feel like they were inadequate, or not worthy of living the life they deserved. I made it my responsibility to make sure that no one around me ever felt these feelings.

Growing up, I was a 'happy go lucky' kid, I took almost everything in stride. My life was completely normal, well I thought so at least. I had an incredibly functional family that molded me into the person I am today. They supported me and guided me. My family made even my wildest dreams come true.

Being the social butterfly I was, I wanted to be friends with everybody. Although that wasn't exactly an attainable goal, I was lucky enough to find a few gems along the way - friends I will have for life. These were the people who got me through the happiest and darkest of days. I think my friends were a large part of the reason I was the kid who jumped out of bed every morning, excited to get to school and see what adventures the day would bring.

School for me was a place where I could express myself, improve myself, and spend plenty of time with my friends. School was where I made most of my fondest memories. It is where I discovered my true potential. I can't sugar coat it too much. Of course there were bad days, and days where I felt the world was coming to an end, but I suppose we all have those days. The fifteen-year-old me, had so many plans and goals for the future. At this point, with the way things were going, they didn't seem too unattainable. I had goals in pretty much everything that I did. I didn't like taking no for an answer.

The Day I Will Never Forget

On the 12th of January 2016, my life took a drastic turn, not one that I could see coming. I had no idea my life would never be the same after that fateful day. All of the goals and future plans I was striving so hard to attain would soon become completely unreachable. You see, that was the day I received my first injection of the HPV vaccine, Gardasil.

But of course, I didn't realize the changes would be so drastic. I actually didn't realize it for a long time. Nothing had changed in my lifestyle. I wasn't doing anything differently but, slowly and surely I felt my body deteriorating. I didn't know why. I started to worry about my body, and how I was feeling. I wasn't okay, but I didn't know why or what was wrong.

It was extremely difficult trying to get help for something I had no idea how to explain. I clearly remember walking into a doctor's office one day and being asked to explain my symptoms. For the first time ever, I sat in front of someone with a mouth full of teeth. I had no idea, I felt like my body was being invaded. I didn't know how, I didn't know why, and I certainly had no idea how to put into words the pain that I was feeling. So, as a result of this I was met with blank stares.

I felt humiliated. My mom and I left the doctor's rooms, and I felt the same, still unable to express what I was feeling. I think the worst part was that the pain was not physically visible. I was the only person that could feel it.

As time progressed my symptoms increased, and so did the pain. I had never been someone that was afraid of much, but for the first time in my life, I was scared. Something was definitely happening. I knew that I wasn't okay. I learned how to explain some of my symptoms, but not all. Even the ones that I could explain rarely made any sense.

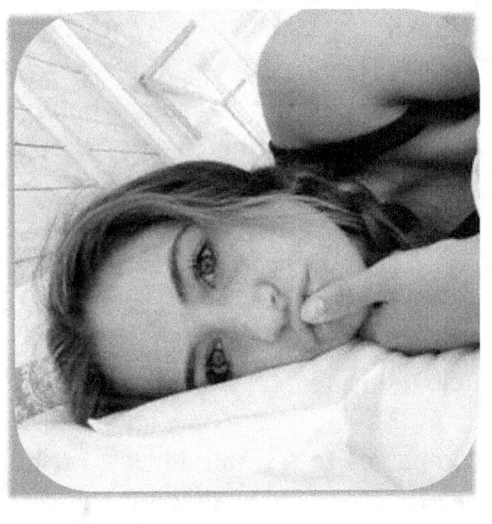

After seeing multiple doctors and specialists, having dozens of tests and scans done, I started to feel helpless. Was I crazy?

I started to question myself and my feelings. I have been told a number of times, that "don't you think that it is psychological?"

Once I was even politely asked to leave the room, so the doctor didn't 'offend' me, whilst telling my mom I needed anti-depressants and it would be a good idea for me to see a psychologist.

Time after time, I was made to feel like a fraud. There was a stage when I was so helpless that I myself started to question whether everything I was feeling was all thought up in my head.

Fast Forward to the Present:

Let's come back to the awards ceremony. I was completely spaced out, consumed with my own thoughts of what could have been. I had always hoped to do great things, whether it was on the sports field, academically, culturally or in the community.

When my body became my worst enemy, I hit rock bottom. Everything I was revolved around the sports I played and the activities I took part in. Now all of that had changed. I found myself at one of the darkest times of my life, purely because of the situation I found myself in. I had always been a problem solver, and suddenly I realized I couldn't solve this one.

I was starting to realize there was no way I could reverse what was happening in my body, and quite frankly neither could anyone else. There are no words that will ever be able to accurately describe the pain, the heartache, and the sense of loss that one feels when this happens.

What I can express is there seems to be no room for people like me in this world, not because I don't belong, but because people don't accept things that make you different.

I do not for one second think what has happened to me is my fault, or my mom's fault. I do however blame the medical fraternity and pharmaceutical companies for their lack of empathy. There are so many unknowns when it comes to this topic. I really do wish for the sake of the person who is sick, that there were more people willing to try and help them.

At the end of the day, you can fight a constant battle against the big companies to try and get justice, but this is nothing compared to the day-to-day battle you fight with yourself.

Although this all sounds like doom and gloom, being sick has given me the opportunity to know and understand myself and my body better than most people.

There is not a moment that goes by when I don't miss the old me. But every now and then, I feel a little bit of appreciation towards the new me. Living in this body is by no means easy, and loving it is even harder. But there are moments when I am grateful for the willpower and the never-ending determination that gets me through the days. There is nothing more powerful than fighting for your life, not against death but against constant trials and tribulations that have the ability to break you down to the inner core.

I am forever grateful that I have had people around me who held me up during times that I didn't think I could stand.

This is the worst kind of illness I could have ever imagined - there is no name, there is no cure, you can't see it, it hides away from the 'usual' blood tests and scans, but it is very much alive. I wish there was something I could say, or something I could do that would make this all better, but I know I can't.

All I can do is take each day as it comes - some days are good, some days are bad, and that's the way my life goes.

Don't get me wrong, there is still so much I am able to enjoy - and now appreciate so much more, like the fact that I can still drink a killer cappuccino with almond milk, or enjoy some delicious gluten free, dairy free cake. Although I am now highly allergic to dairy and gluten, and seriously miss things like ice-cream and a good hot chocolate, I have managed to find some good alternatives.

I miss living a carefree life but being sick has taught me how to listen to my body and rely on it completely. It has taught me to love myself, because in a flash, it can all be taken away. I think I take my broken body for granted sometimes and push it a little too far. But I think every day you slowly learn what is good and what is not.

Things like hot classrooms, or buildings, high intensity sporting activities, stuffy areas, and airports - and if I thought being hot was bad, being cold is just as bad; the countless hours spent trying to warm my hypothermic body up after being in the cold; or my hands that go numb because there is no blood circulation; or even how my legs turn blue and don't return to their normal color without a nice warm bath. All of these silly things play such a huge role in who I am now.

So next time you look at me, I know you will see the girl that has brown hair, blue eyes, and is slightly curved but take a little time to think that that girl you see, the one that looks like she has it all together, is also the girl that really doesn't.

My Future?

I am Shaina Wheeler, and this is my story. Looking back at the journey I have embarked on over the last two years brings a tear to my eye. When I was younger, I pictured how I would start my final year of school. I did not picture this. Keep reading, it's probably not what you think.

I always thought I would be the girl who started her final year problem free, except for the typical school shenanigans, of course. Well, problem free is very far from me. I never really envisioned bags of medications and countless trips to the nurse's office. Little did I know I would be best friends with some of the staff because I gave them a free gym workout for the day because I had fainted somewhere around school. Now friends have to pick me up and carry me to the nurse. Yes, not really the picture I had in mind.

Would I change things? Sure, it would be great not to have to go through these challenges on a daily basis. But, not for a second would I change my journey. Not for a second would I wish that this had never happened to me. I am a firm believer in the fact that everything happens for a reason. Cliché, I know.

You may be wondering why I'm writing this. It's because today is the anniversary for me – today is two years since my life got turned completely upside down. Two years ago I received the HPV vaccine Gardasil.

So, this is me - I am Shaina Wheeler, and I am an eighteen-year-old girl, whose life was drastically changed by the HPV vaccine. There is a song, from one of my favorite films, *The Greatest Showman*, called '*This is me*'. This is my theme song, it talks about the feeling of being undesirable, not being good enough for this world and the journey toward self-acceptance and how one learns not to be ashamed of themselves, and to rather be proud of everything that you've overcome.

I really am a strong believer in the saying that everything happens for a reason. I don't enjoy my teenage years being stolen from me, or that my body became my worst enemy. But this entire journey has shown me that I can overcome anything that is put in my way. It is difficult to think I will never go back to being the person I once was. I will never be a sportswoman, but it does humble me to think about how much my life has changed and all of the new opportunities that I have been faced with.

I used to live by the motto "Don't wait for the storm to pass, learn to dance in the rain."

Unfortunately, the rain soaked me, and I had to alter my motto a bit.

My new motto is:

"Don't wait for the storm to pass; learn to dance with the rain."

Looking back at the girl from two years ago on this day, I wish there was a way I could somehow warn her about all the struggles she is about to face. I wish I could warn her about all the pain, disbelief, heartbreak and uncertainty that lies ahead. I wish I could tell her to be strong. I wish I could tell her to be strong, to tell her that she will be okay in the end and that even though she wants to give up, she will make it. She can do it.

If I could write a letter to me in 2016, this is what I would say:

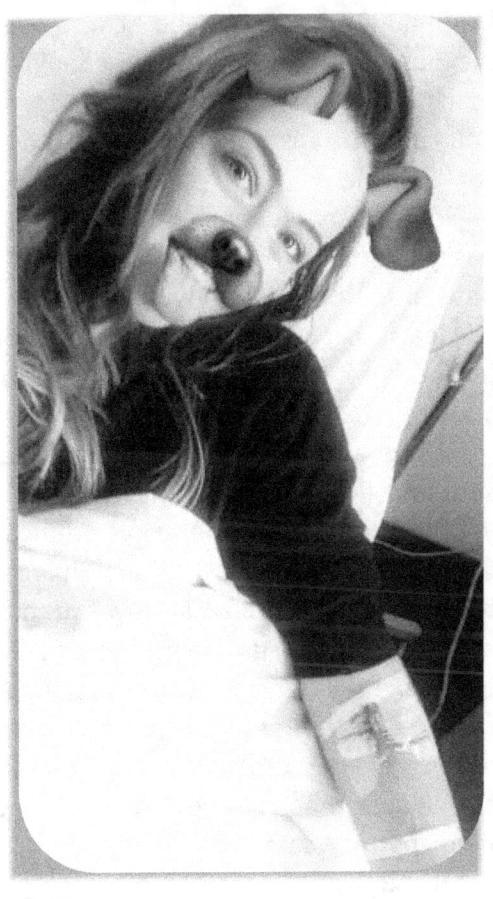

Hey Shay,

This is you, from the future... I need you to listen, and I need you to listen carefully. What is about to happen is going to feel surreal, you're going to feel confused. You're going to feel sick, all the time, you're not going to know why. You're not going to know how to explain it.

You're going to feel nauseous constantly. You are going to lose feeling of your right arm. But don't worry, you're going to be okay. You will teach yourself how to use it again. At first you'll drop things, you'll be scared and cry and scream, you'll be frustrated, but then you'll soon teach yourself how to write again. It will be hard, but you can do it. Your arm will constantly shake, doctors will do tests but you'll never get an answer. Don't question yourself. You are not alone.

You'll be put on thousands of medications. Just breathe. Trust the process, you're going to be okay in the end, and if it's not okay then it's not the end. Take the medications, but trust yourself, you know your body and you know what's right for you.

You will have doctors and people that tell you that it is all in your head. It's okay to cry when this happens - you will realize that it is not all in your head, and as frustrated as you will be, you'll learn that those doctors wouldn't have been able to help you anyway.

You know the truth and you know how you feel, or at least you will start to understand it after a while. You will become a regular at the hospital - it's okay to be scared, but they will love you. You'll be diagnosed with some pretty hectic illnesses - it's okay. I promise, they teach you a lot. They are difficult to understand, difficult to deal with. You can't run from them, so please don't try. There is nothing that you can't handle.

You will hate yourself for a bit - only because you want to be everything that you were before. It will take you a while to adjust to the new you. A part of you will never fully accept this new person, but you will learn that she is actually pretty cool.

You don't need to blame yourself for what has happened or for how you feel, that is not going to help you. Stay positive you'll be alright.

School will be the penultimate test. You will feel let down, it's something that you will have to embrace. You will feel like you let yourself down, even though you almost killed yourself in the process of trying to be something great. Change your goals, you used to be so focused on succeeding, shift your focus to surviving, anything over and above...Well baby girl, makes you a star.

People will let you down, teachers will let you down, friends, and family - but don't sweat the small stuff. Nobody understands, not even you. Your symptoms will never be understood fully, not by you, not by the people that love you, nor the people that have the capability to help you. As I said before - trust the process, it's the only way you will get through each day.

When you look in the mirror Shay - don't be surprised when you don't see the same eyes, the same smile, or the same body. You are different now, but different does not mean ugly, fat, or withered. It will break your heart if you look into the mirror hoping to see those super sporty legs, or those shining eyes - please do remember those eyes glittered like that before because they had never been exposed to chronic pain. Now they tell a story, a story more beautiful and more meaningful than any other you have ever told before. Look at the new, beautiful girl you see staring back. Embrace this. Trust me.

I wish you knew how hard it is going to be and I wish I could prepare you. But I know nothing will. Nothing will prepare you for the sleepless nights, the nights that you cry yourself to sleep in the hospital beds, the nights you scream in pain, and the nights you are so sore you felt nothing at all.

I'm so sorry.

Please know that you are okay in the end.

Push hard.

Use every inch of strength you've got.

You are great.

So yes if I were to write a letter that is what it would say. Because nothing could ever prepare someone for the constant headaches that feel like a nail is going into your head, or the nausea that makes you feel like you're being punched in the stomach, or the random fainting that is so uncontrollable. The best part is that people think it's an act.

Do they really think if I had a choice I would choose to be in pain 24/7?

Sitting here writing this right now I can only be grateful that I am here now and not where I was two years ago. It has been a long, and

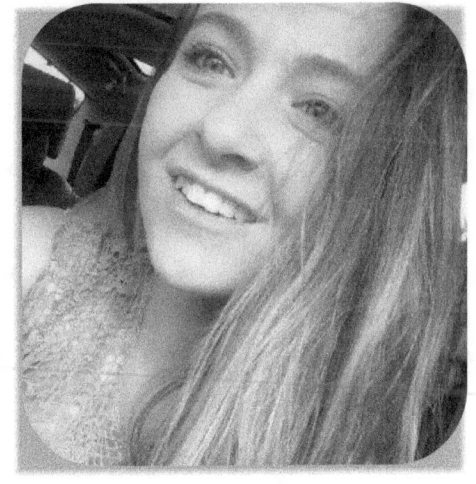

excruciating road to get to where I am today. The journey is so far from over. But I'm also two years more knowledgeable than I was.

There have been times I have felt so low, that I wondered if all of this was worth it? Is fighting for this broken body worth it at all? I often wondered to myself if I was fighting because I wanted to or because I felt like I should for the 'cause.'

After countless debates with myself I came to the realization that I was given this for a reason. I don't know what that reason is yet, but there is a reason.

I would love to have my old life back. Be a competitive showjumper and eventer. Play every sport under the sun. Be the girl I talk about in stories. I mean sure, I would love to get back to that but that's not me anymore.

Right now I've embraced this journey and I'm making the most of it because there is beauty in all things. I want you all to know a broken body does not mean a broken spirit.

And if you see me out and about looking very normal I'll take the compliment and thank painkillers for that one, and I'll be grateful that I was able to make it out of the house to wherever I was. My life is by no means normal.

We keep it interesting in the Wheeler household. Always keeping you on your toes. Keeping it real. It's a tough day for me so I'm trying to hold it together. I'm sorry if this was very strange and disjointed. Just thought I'd share how I felt about one of the hardest days of my living existence.

So on this day, I'm going to smile and keep pushing because after all, I'm on this journey and giving up is not part of my plan!

CHAPTER 6

Central and South America

Costa Rica

Costa Rica is evidently one of the go-to places for conducting clinical trials. In the early 1990's the United States government Public Health Services provided research support for the Guanacaste Project. The Guanacaste province of Costa Rica is rural and had a consistently high rate of invasive cervical cancer. The primary purpose of the study was to investigate the role of human papillomavirus and its co-factors in the development of high-grade cervical lesions. Over 10,000 women over the age of 18 were enrolled in the initial study. A comprehensive physical exam at the beginning of the study was to serve as a baseline for measuring against data obtained from following the women over several years. Anyone free from serious disease would be followed up with on a regular basis to study the natural history of HPV infections. The hope was that by conducting regular visual, microscopic, molecular, and serological testing they could characterize the natural history of HPV infections and the origin of high-grade cervical lesions.[126]

Somewhere along the line, the research population dropped from 10,000 to only 6,000. Perhaps some were lost to follow-up over such a

---

[126] Herrero, R., Schiffman, MH, Bratti, C., et al; Design and methods of a population-based study of cervical neoplasia in a rural province of Costa Rica: the Guanacaste Project; May 1997; PMID 9180057

long period of time. Or, perhaps the women who developed serious diseases were dropped from the study cohort.

From 1992 through 2000, this project was funded by no less than 22 grants from the United States NIH (National Institute of Health). The grants were approximately $1.4 million each.[127]

Costa Rica had instituted a national plan for the detection of cervical cancer in 1960. The plan was carried out at family planning visits and used cervical/vaginal cytology. Between 1965 and 1980, cervical cancer mortality was reduced by more than half and the rate of diagnosis went from 50/100,000 to 36/100,000. Due to Costa Rica's ongoing commitment to cervical cancer prevention, both rates continued to drop over the next two decades.[128]

An article published in the *BMJ* (British Medical Journal) described another clinical trial in Guanacaste, Costa Rica. The trial would be conducted in seven clinics with 7,466 participants divided into two groups. One would receive 3 doses of Cervarix and the other would be injected with a three-dose formulation of the hepatitis A vaccine, Twinrix.[129]

When women between the ages of 18 and 25 were interviewed for participation in this trial, they were excluded if they had any of the following conditions:

- Chronic disease
- A history of severe allergic reactions to vaccines
- A history of hepatitis A, or previous vaccination against it
- A history of the chronic administration of immunosuppressive drugs
- A history of immunosuppressive conditions
- Hysterectomy
- The use of other investigative products in the last 30 days
- Previous administration of the ASO4 adjuvant

---

[127] Bratti, Conception C.; Guanacaste Project-A Population Based Natural Hist; NIH Grantome; accessed March 2019

[128] Ileana Quiros Rojas; The cervical cancer prevention programme in Costa Rica; 8 Oct 2015; PMID 26557876

[129] Herrero, Rolando et al. "Rationale and design of a community-based double-blind randomized clinical trial of an HPV 16 and 18 vaccine in Guanacaste, Costa Rica." *Vaccine* vol. 26, 37 (2008): 4795-808. doi:10.1016/j.vaccine.2008.07.002; PMID 18640170

- Previous HPV vaccination
- Allergy to 2 phenoxy-methanol or neomycin
- Latex sensitivity
- An unwillingness to use contraception as per protocol
- Pregnant or less than 3 months post-partum
- Currently lactating
- Any acute condition expected to resolve soon
- Recent administration of a vaccine or immunoglobulin

Of the 7,466 original participants, one was excluded for receiving the wrong vaccine at one of her visits. Of the remaining 7,465 participants, 5,988 got 3 doses, 928 participants missed 1 dose. Of those who missed a dose, the reasons are as follows:

- 302 (32.5%) pregnancy
- 192 (20.7%) missed visit
- 145 (15.6%) medical condition
- 120 (12.9%) refusal of dose
- 27 (2.9%) referred to colposcopy
- 142 (15.3%) other reasons

In October 2011, *The Journal of the National Cancer Institute*, published a re-analysis of the data from the study referred to above. The conclusion of this analysis stated, "Four years after vaccination of women who appeared to be uninfected, this nonrandomized analysis suggests that two doses of the HPV16/18 vaccine, and maybe even one dose, are as protective as three doses."[130]

In September of 2011, Aimee Kreimer, PhD, prepared a PowerPoint presentation that revealed the actual results of this analysis.[131] The results she presented are as follows:

- Efficacy in those who received 3 doses was 80.9%
- Efficacy in those who received 2 doses was 84.1%

---

[130] Kreimer, Aimee R, PhD, et al; Proof-of-Principle Evaluation pf the Efficacy pf Fewer Than Three Doses of a Bivalent HPV16/18 Vaccine; Journal of the National Cancer Institute, Volume 103; Issue 19, Pages 1444-1451; 5 Oct 2011; PMID 21908768

[131] Kreimer, Aimee, PhD; Recent Findings from the NCI Costa Rica HPV-16/18 Vaccine Trial; NCI,USDHHS, NIH; PowerPoint Presentation; accessed March 2019

- Efficacy in those who received 1 dose was 100%

Considering this information was known in 2011, one has to wonder why most of the world is still promoting either two or three doses of HPV vaccines.

16 October 2017, Costa Rica's National Immunization Technical Advisory Group (NITAG) recommended the introduction of the rotavirus and human papillomavirus vaccines to the national immunization program. The rotavirus would be included in the next year's immunization program. It was estimated that the HPV vaccine could be added to the national immunization program in 2019.[132]

In 2019, Costa Rica announced that 20,000 adolescents between the ages of 12 and 16 would be vaccinated with HPV vaccine as part of yet another research project. The vaccination program would be administered in a two-dose schedule with injections six months apart. The invitation to participate would be extended to girls in Guanacaste and other cantons. Evidently some participants were to receive one dose and others two because the participants in this trial were scheduled to be followed for four years in order to determine whether one dose was as effective as two or three doses.[133]

---

[132] NITAG Resource Center; 16 Oct 2007; accessed March 2019
[133] Staff writer; 20 thousand teenagers will be vaccinated against human papillomavirus; Diario Extra; 25 March 2019; accessed March 2019

Doctor's Advice Left Me Paralyzed

Submitted by Mario Lamo-Jiménez

Laura Navarro Calvo is a 29-year-old Costa Rican woman who received the Gardasil vaccine in 2014. She was never advised about the side effects of the vaccine and wasn't provided with an informed consent form to sign. She was only told that the vaccine was applied to 'prevent cervical cancer' and became paralyzed 24 hours after receiving the first dose.

Laura is currently disabled. According to her doctors, there isn't any treatment for her illness and the damage is irreversible. The Costa Rican government doesn't recognize that the vaccine causes any damage.

She says that the government:

> "Should report that the real side effects of this vaccine go beyond arm pain or dizziness. It reduced my life to receiving therapies, to going to doctors' appointments, and to being confined to a wheelchair. There have been thousands of cases in the world like mine where the vaccine has caused much damage, it has destroyed people's lives."

This is her story, in her own words.

"I had come back from a trip to Nicaragua, so I went to my medical appointment, as I always do once a year. I went to my doctor's office, and after the routine examinations that are performed the doctor advised me to get vaccinated against HPV as a preventive measure. He informed me that it was a good thing to do since I was also near the age limit to get vaccinated, which was 25 years of age. I got vaccinated and returned home. I felt some pain in my arm, but it was normal, like with any other injection, or so I thought.

The first day passed. I went to sleep, and the next day I woke up with pain in my legs and with pain in my lower back. I was so tired that I fell asleep again. When I tried to get out of bed, I couldn't, I felt that my legs were completely paralyzed, and from that moment on, I could never walk normally again.

I went to the emergency room of the Heredia Hospital, where they performed several tests on me, and treated me for chikungunya (a mosquito-borne illness) since I had been out of the country. But it was never confirmed that I had that illness.

I left the hospital and went home without any diagnosis. I had several laboratory studies done until I found an internist, an infectious disease doctor, who was the one that referred me to the Mexican Hospital for some neurological studies, with a possible diagnosis of Guillain-Barre. At the Mexican Hospital I was admitted through the emergency department where they performed studies such as a CAT scan and lab tests. They also performed a lumbar puncture which **showed** that the fluid was affected so I was admitted as a possible Guillain-Barre case.

By then, my legs were completely paralyzed. The internist noted that I had inflammation of the brain, a partial paralysis of my face and I also had acute pain. The vaccine was the only thing that they were able to associate with my illnesses after the medical exams, since I had been completely healthy and everything began after the vaccine.

I suffer headaches, I have cramps, tingling, vomiting. I have a loss of control of the sphincter. I had memory loss. I have lost my sense of direction. I basically don't sleep. I go through very bad nights. There are many adverse effects that I suffer every day.

Before the vaccine I was very normal. I worked and I studied. I also knew several languages, which is knowledge that I have lost, I suppose for the same reason, (the vaccine) and I haven't been able to recover that knowledge. I used to travel, to play soccer, to swim, to run. I had a full life that was completely normal for a person of my age, but now everything has been totally altered.

Previously, I lived by myself, I was fully independent in my own apartment; I had my own car. Everything was normal. But now, I have had to come back to live with my parents since they are taking care of me economically and medically. They are with me every single day. This has been a very abrupt change in my life because I can't perform the simple task of walking. That has made a huge difference for me."

Colombia

Gardasil in Colombia: An Introduction

By Mario Lamo-Jiménez

The vaccine against HPV was introduced in Colombia in 2013 in a strange fashion: Congress created a law (Law 1626, approved on April 30, 2013) stating that vaccination against HPV was 'free and mandatory for the target population.'[134]

Vaccination without informed consent

In 2013, the Colombian government spent close to a hundred million dollars on HPV vaccines and started the National Gardasil Vaccination Campaign. Neither the families nor the vaccinated girls had a word to say about it. The 'target population' barely knew what the vaccine was being used for. Not even the manufacturer's information about the possible side effects of the vaccine was provided to anyone.

There was no informed consent. Since the law stated that all girls starting at 9 years of age had to be vaccinated, the Ministry of Health set a vaccination quota that had to be filled.

This was a law enacted by politicians. The full Congress approved the law. No one opposed it, although most members of Congress didn't really know what they were voting on.

In 2014 I had the opportunity to personally tell one of the Colombian senators who had voted for the law about how the vaccine was causing terrible side effects in many young girls. He said that he didn't know about the matter, but promised me that somebody from his staff would look into it. Now, five years later, I still have not heard back from him.

---

[134] Publicada en el Diario Oficial 48777 de abril 30 de 2013; accessed April 2019

Mass side effects: Carmen de Bolívar: A tragedy foretold

In 2012, I had returned to Colombia after living for decades in the US. The following year on February 2013, I saw a newspaper article stating that:

The government wanted to vaccinate three-and-a-half million girls who were attending school. Many were below reproductive age.[135]

I was outraged by this information! I knew Gardasil had caused harm in the States and several other countries in the world.

I feared the same thing was going to happen in Colombia. So, I wrote a blog article discussing the dangers of the HPV vaccine and submitted it to a major Colombian newspaper, *El Tiempo*. The article was censored by this, the largest paper in Colombia. They accused me of spreading false information and I was told that Merck was going to sue me. So, I sent the paper a second article including more than 50 pages of extensive references backing up every single fact stated in my original article. Instead of publishing the second piece with references, they closed my blog and deleted my original article.[136]

The current situation in Carmen de Bolívar

There are already more than a thousand cases of girls in Carmen de Bolívar reporting symptoms of fainting, shortness of breath and weakness in the limbs. What do these girls have in common? All received Gardasil, a vaccine that supposedly helps prevent cervical cancer, which they say may be caused by the human papillomavirus.

The government emphatically denies that the vaccine is causing these symptoms.[137] However, the parents of these affected girls disagree.

For the first time in the history of Colombia, and perhaps of the world, there is massive protest because of a vaccine that is apparently making people sick instead of protecting them.

---

[135] Writing Life Today; All high school graduates will receive the human papillomavirus vaccine; El Tiempo; 21 Jan 2013; accessed April 2019

[136] Mario Lamo-Jiménez; Gardasil, the Vaccine that Kills; republished Alliance of Writers and Journalists; accessed April 2019

[137] Living Writing; 'The HPV vaccine is safe'; El Espectador; 26 Aug 2014; accessed April 2019

Some family members have staged peaceful protest marches to demand immediate investigations; others burned tires in protest and blocked a main road that connects a coastal town of Colombia with the interior of the country.[138]

According to a local teacher, the girls in Carmen de Bolivar received their first dose of Gardasil in July 2013 after which reported reactions were similar to other vaccines such as redness, swelling, pain at the injection site, etc. When the second dose was administered on the 20th of March 2014, several girls reacted immediately and much more severely, reporting dizziness, fainting, and severe headaches. By May 29th and 30th, the situation had turned into a full-blown crisis with scores of girls being admitted to local emergency room facilities to be treated for fainting, shortness of breath, and weakness in the limbs among other symptoms.[139]

The victims carried signs with their demands and grievances:

- WE WANT SOLUTIONS!
- VACCINES THAT KILL ARE ORGANIZED CRIME.
- BIG PHARMA CORRUPTS THE HEALTH SYSTEM.
- CARMEN DE BOLÍVAR IS OUTRAGED.
- WE WANT HEALTHY GIRLS WITHOUT THE SIDE EFFECTS OF THE HPV VACCINE.
- MASS PSYCHOGENIC ILLNESS AT THE MINISTRY OF HEALTH BECAUSE OF THE 400 GIRLS VICTIMS OF THE VACCINE AGAINST HPV.

The Government's Answer:

- The Minister of Health has threatened critics with legal actions.
- The Minister of Health has dismissed legal actions by victims saying the lawyers want to get rich.
- The Minister of Health has said that in Colombia scientific facts are decided by tribunals.

---

[138] Vicente Arcieri; Parents of girls from Carmen de Bolivar block school entranced; El Heraldo; 11 July 2016; accessed April 2019

[139] Mario Lamo-Jiménez; Vaccine against HPV: announced tragedy; Los 2 Orillas; 28 Aug 2014; accessed April 2019

- The Minister of Health has said that the Gardasil vaccine, contrary to all evidence, is perfectly safe.
- The Minister of Health has said that side effects of the Gardasil vaccine are a case of 'massive hysteria.'
- The Minister of Health was an Engineer and an Economist, a political appointee with no health-related degrees.

After the scandal in Carmen de Bolívar, Gardasil vaccination rates in Colombia went down to a meager 5%. The victims still aren't receiving proper treatment.

The victims of the vaccine and their families have had more than 200 meetings with government representatives who had offered to help. They have signed several agreements to do so. For example, one offered an ambulance so the girls who live in hard-to-access parts of the municipality could be taken to the hospital when they were having seizures. But, not one single one of these government promises has been fulfilled. They didn't even provide the ambulance.

Thanks to a lawsuit, the Gardasil vaccine stopped being mandatory in Colombia in 2017 and a court of law established the need for 'informed consent' to administer the vaccine.[140]

A lawsuit was filed in Colombia against Merck in 2017 alleging that the Gardasil vaccine was unsafe and that it had caused many victims with various syndromes. The lawsuit is currently pending.[141]

Update:

In January of this year 2019, I had the opportunity to travel to Carmen de Bolívar, a small Colombian town near the Caribbean Sea where I was able to interview some of the victims and their parents. The victims of the vaccine aren't receiving any treatment. Three young women have died. Dozens of others have tried to commit suicide because they don't see their situation improving and realize that their quality of life is in fact deteriorating.

---

[140] Constitutional Court Record; Judgment T-365/17; Bogota DC; 2 June 2017; accessed April 2019

[141] Mario Lamo-Jiménez; Claim for $160 million dollsrs against Merch for damages caused by the Gardasil vaccine in Colombia; Las 2 Orillas; 18 Aug 2017; accessed April 2019

Many families have had to sell their belongings in order to obtain alternative treatments for their daughters. So far, none of the girls have been cured.

The government produced a study in 2018 saying that the girls 'were sick and needed urgent treatment,' but that they 'didn't know what the cause of their illnesses was.'

Currently the affected girls don't have any diagnosis since the government vehemently denies that the vaccine caused any damage. Therefore, there isn't any treatment protocol that is being followed for the multiple afflictions that they are presenting.[142]

Here are some of the symptoms experienced by the girls in Carmen de Bolívar, according to a survey conducted by Dr. Pompillio Martínez:

> "Headaches, Leg pain, Asphyxia, choking, dyspnea, Chest pain, Tingling of legs, Tingling of hands or arms, Weakness/Low muscle strength, Changes of mood, Weight changes, Fatigue, Palpitations, Weakness or loss of leg muscle strength, Leg stiffness or cramping, Loss of leg sensitivity, hand pain, Interference with school activities, homework,

> Neck pain, Difficulty walking, Stiffness or cramping in arms, Pain in the foot, Loss of arms' sensitivity, Leg tremors, Fever, chills, sweating, Muscle Pain in the Legs, Dizziness (vertigo), Spinal column pain, Dizziness (fainting, syncope, pale), Tremors in the arms, Changes in concentration, Dizziness (nausea with or without vomiting), Loss of consciousness, Hair loss, Flaccidity or muscle atrophy in the arms, Changes in menstruation, Flaccidity or muscle atrophy in the legs, Difficulty in articulating words, Insomnia, Urinary incontinence, Susceptibility to infections, Difficulty eating or drinking, Diarrhea, Bruises on the body, Bleeding nasal or gums, Armpit pain, Fecal incontinence."[143]

---

[142] Biweekly National Epidemiological Report; Bogota DC Volume 20 No 3-4; Feb 2015; accessed April 2019

[143] Pompillio Martinez, MD; Survey analysis of affected symptoms of Carmen de Bolivar; 8 July 2015; accessed April 2019

Carmen de Bolívar has had a history of violence. Almost twenty years ago, very many of the inhabitants of a neighboring small town were massacred by paramilitary groups. Many people just left their land and their houses, since the objective of the paramilitary groups was to obtain the land for the big landowners and they did so.[144]

People had just started returning to the area, especially after a peace treaty with the largest insurgent group in Colombia, FARC, was signed in 2016. Things were starting to settle down. Families had regrouped and were beginning to plow what was left of their land once more... and then the National Gardasil Vaccination Campaign came. It was like being struck by lightning twice. This time the assault was not perpetrated by armed paramilitary men, but by the government itself with women armed with syringes.

The vaccine is basically destroying the social fabric of a community that was still recovering from an intense degree of violence perpetrated by paramilitary groups.

The first interview that you will read here was conducted with María José Blanco Cárdenas in the town of El Salado, the very same place where paramilitary groups murdered more than a hundred people from the 16-22 of February 2000.

The second one was conducted with Rosa Salina in a place called 'La Cansona,' which literally means in Spanish 'The tiresome one,' since to get there you have to take a road that goes uphill and you get very tired walking all the way there. Rosa Salina is a very articulate 18-year old who narrates with many details how the vaccine basically changed her life and the life of her family, shattering many dreams. In spite of everything, she has maintained her resilience and her intellect. She trusts that one day she will overcome the harm the vaccine has caused her.

---

[144] Rochter, Larry; Colombians Tell of massacre, as Army Stood By; The New York Times; 14 July 2000; accessed April 2019

Interview with María José Blanco Cárdenas

El Salado, January 22nd, 2019, 12:08 pm

My name is María José Blanco Cárdenas, we are now in El Salado, Bolívar. I was vaccinated at the Holy Spirit Educational Institute. I was about 14 or 15 years old when I was vaccinated. The experience that I have had with the vaccine has been terrible. I have gone to many clinics. I have had many crises. The crises appear in different forms. For example, sometimes I completely lose the ability 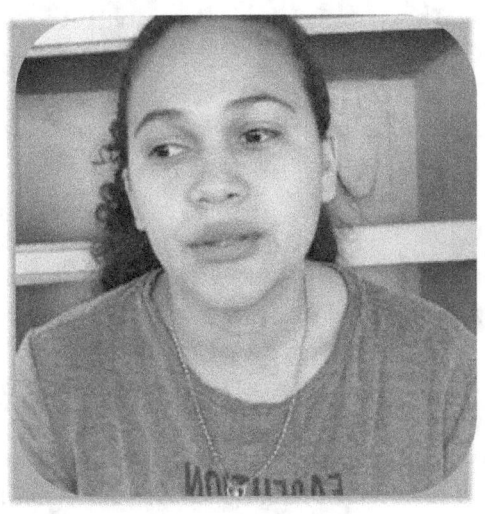 to move my legs, or I sleep for almost 24 hours and I don't awaken no matter how they try to wake me up.

The truth is that I have been suffering a lot because of this. There have been opportunities that I have missed because of the pains I suffer. I have become the butt of the jokes of many people. I have also felt the pain that my family feels when they see me in this condition, when they see how I feel, the reactions I have.

This hasn't been easy because I have missed many opportunities that I couldn't take advantage of since I was sick, because I was in a clinic, on a stretcher, where doctors have never told me what I really have.

I have wanted to kill myself because I don't want to be like this anymore; because I see how my family suffers when they see me ill and knowing that we are still without finding a solution. I want to move ahead with my life but I haven't been able to. Instead I suffer like many other girls.

I'm afraid that one day I will fall asleep and will never wake up, or that I will be bound to a wheelchair without knowing why this happened. This is a lumbar pain, a regular pain, that is what the doctors have said, but I don't feel it that way. It hurts. I'm feeling it. I want this to end. I want to know what it is that I have. I want a solution for my health. I want this to end...

How many times were you vaccinated?

They came to inject me with the third dose. I had the third dose of that vaccine, and because of that I'm going through very ugly things.

Did you have any symptoms with the first dose?

With the first dose I didn't feel anything or maybe I didn't notice. With the second dose I started to feel everything. My body started to react in a different way. With the third dose everything really started and they didn't even ask for any consent from my parents.

Were you told what the vaccine was for?

They said it was against the human papilloma virus and we got vaccinated at school, but that was everything we were told.

Were you told of any risks associated with the vaccine?

No, they didn't tell us about any risks, they said it was for our health for our well-being. But now I can see what the "well-being" was that we were injected with.

This has affected my life because I have wanted to study. But in spite of that wish, I have fallen behind, because I have sometimes been in the hospital suffering with pain. It has affected my family in the way that I see them destroyed when they see me like this. The little they have, or had, they have sold it and they are in debt because they have been trying to find a medical solution for me; taking me to clinics, looking for an answer and not finding one.

Are you receiving any treatment right now?

No, I'm not receiving any type of treatment, only when I go to the hospital because of the pain. They inject me with some medicine, give me some pills and with that I have to stand the pain. Everything that happens, with a few pills because I am not receiving any treatment.

They don't tell me anything because according to them, they don't know what my illness is.

What are the stronger symptoms that you feel?

The strongest pain that I have had is a pain in my spine, a lumbar pain that affects me all over, even in my legs. I stop feeling my legs. I can't move them. They do not respond to anything, to any stimulation. It is very painful just to think that I may become wheelchair bound and that I may not be able to walk again because of this.

Have you received any diagnosis?

They don't give me any diagnosis.

Have you had any tests done?

Yes, they have done many tests.

What have the tests shown?

They have told me that it is just a lumbar pain that can go away with an injection. They have told me that it is a normal type of infection that can be treated with antibiotics, and that is it.

This only offers you a temporary help?

Yes, it is something temporary.

Are there stronger episodes where you feel weaker?

Yes, I have episodes when I sleep for almost 24 hours, I don't respond to any type of stimulus. When I wake up, I'm not able to be awake for a long time, it is like my body is just tired and only wants to sleep and to rest. My body doesn't want to respond and I don't even move at all.

Were you able to continue with your studies?

No, it has been difficult. No matter how much I want to feel better, I even made the decision to not continue. I stopped seeking more doctors or going to clinics, but decided instead to struggle for my dream of wanting to study, of going ahead with my life. If I feel pain I endure it, but I want to study, I want to move ahead.

What expectations do you have now after talking with the Attorney General?

I have the expectation that perhaps something will be solved, because I was able to talk to him and I was able to see that he paid attention to me. He listened to me, that he indeed felt the message I wanted to convey to him and I hope that he will help us, that this time we will indeed be heard.

Did he make any promises?

He didn't commit himself directly to looking for a solution. But I know that he is going to help us; that he is going to try. I hope he will be heard, so they can see that what we are feeling is real and that we need help.

What do you feel when the papers publish news articles saying that nothing happened here, that everybody is well?

I don't know if I feel anger or disappointment. This indeed happened, because of what we are feeling. It happened because we are enduring this, not only us, but our families also. I'm very mad when they say that nothing happened here when the real situation is not like that. Why do they try to hide the facts if we are the ones who are feeling ill?

What would you say to other girls who may be thinking about getting this vaccine?

I would think about it and I wouldn't get vaccinated. The ones that indeed got vaccinated are the example and we are suffering. The girls who are going to be vaccinated should think about it; should talk with their parents and should be aware at the moment of vaccination. We cannot even trust the vaccination. They should first prove to them that this is not going to happen to them; that they are not going to go through the same things that so many girls are enduring.

You were vaccinated in Carmen...

Yes, I was vaccinated in Carmen de Bolívar.

But you are from El Salado...

I live here.

But you were attending school in Carmen de Bolívar.

Yes, I was attending school in Carmen de Bolívar.

Thank you very much, good luck.

Thank you.

Interview with Rosa Salinas

La Cansona, Carmen de Bolívar, Colombia, Jan 23rd, 2019 3:04 pm

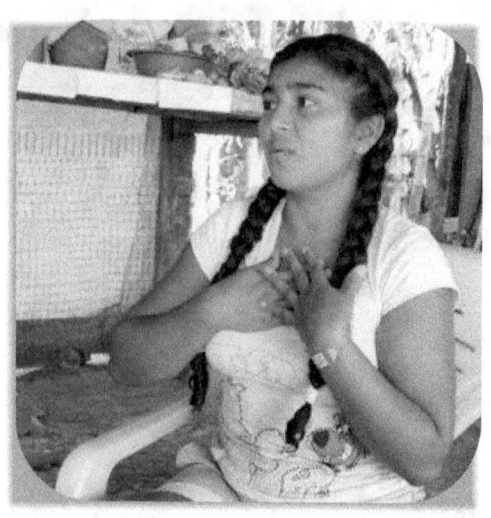

Well, my name is Rosa Salinas and I'm 18 years old. I already completed high school and I live in the municipality of La Cansona. I'm currently studying a technical career in Early Childhood Education. I live with my parents, and beginning on September 12th, 2014, the crises started.

They started vaccinating at my school, one of my schoolmates fainted and I helped her, but after that my body lost its strength. I fainted too. I was taken to the hospital, I was completely unconscious. Many of my schoolmates were taken along with me, in just one car. Many girls were arriving with their mothers. My mother was here up on the mountain and I was at school, which is in a lower municipality.

The teachers called my mother, and when she arrived I started crying. I was very frightened because this was something that I had seen but never thought would happen to me. I never thought that I would faint. I only observed what was happening and would tell my mom. "A classmate fainted." But I never thought that it would happen to me too. But then, I was vaccinated as well.

What happened after the first dose or the second one?

It was after the second dose. Sincerely, I didn't try to resist it. "We are going to vaccinate you against cervical cancer," I was told. Fine. Some of my classmates resisted it. They said "No!"

They ran away, kicked their legs, but the teachers grabbed them, and they surrendered to the vaccine. One of my classmates who resisted the vaccine was vaccinated. She had a crisis about two times.

After that she had a skin eruption. She stopped wearing shorts; she wouldn't wear short clothing. She would only wear long clothing, like jeans. She hasn't had any more crises, but she has a skin problem, which is an effect of the vaccine on the skin.

I have prayed to God; I have asked God to help me. I consider myself in a certain sense a courageous person. I like to study; I like children. That is why I'm studying early childhood education. My goals are to move out of here, to continue studying, to be a professional...

I try day-to-day to live with this. Yes, this is a true disease and it is uncomfortable when I want to study but I can't because my head hurts too much, because I'm dizzy, because my legs hurt and there are pains that come and go. I feel normal, I'm fine, I'm jumping, I'm playing, then I feel that my chest hurts. I'm out of breath, my leg hurts, that I cannot do things because my head hurts, that I might fall down. These are very uncomfortable situations for us, for me, well, certainly for me.

In the place I am studying now, in the university, I haven't had a crisis. But, after arriving here at home I have had them. And it's dangerous because I come on my motorcycle. My means of transportation is the motorcycle. If I get a crisis while on the motorcycle, I might fall off and die in the road. This is something uncertain, because the crises can happen at any time.

How did this change your life, the fact of having these symptoms, have you felt tired? How is your learning now?

When I was studying in high school, when this started in ninth grade, I stopped going to school. It was a big decision that I had to make, because at the beginning I was fainting every day. The pains were constant, and they gave me pills. It seemed like my body couldn't stand any more pills, they took me to the hospital and they treated me very inhumanely, like: "Look at her, she needs a man or something else."

During that period of time when I was at home, not going to school, I almost didn't pass the 9th grade; I have always passed every school year. I have always finished what I started, no matter what. In the middle of the school year, they told me that I wasn't doing well. I told my mother that this couldn't be happening, and against all odds I was able to recover; and thank God I did well that year, in spite of everything.

It is uncomfortable to be like this, but I have had to resign myself and learn to live with this situation.

When you were vaccinated, did they explain what the vaccine was for, what the virus is, did you receive any paper listing the possible side effects the vaccine could have?

No, no. They came to the classroom and said that on that day they were going to vaccinate against cervical cancer which had killed many women and that was it. They didn't tell us that the vaccine could cause dizziness, headache, that we could faint, or that you wouldn't feel well, no.

They just said, "It is just one more vaccine; this will help you with your life, allow yourselves to be vaccinated."

Some of my classmates didn't want to receive the vaccine and they were told by the teachers: "Either you get vaccinated or you will fail the course or will fail the year with me."

I said to myself, "Okay, I won't fail a school year for not letting them vaccinate me." I showed them my arm and they vaccinated me. As simple as that.

At the beginning I didn't feel anything. Everything was normal. But later, my legs were affected. I felt like I was going to fall. My chest was affected, my breathing, I felt like I was choking, then I completely lost consciousness and fell to the ground. My classmates told me that I was put into a car with other classmates. There were a lot of girls that time almost all of the girls of Caracolí, our town, fainted.

Was that with the second dose?

Yes. It wasn't with the first one... but there was one particular case while I was studying there, there was a girl who fainted and fainted. She finished school and I haven't heard anything else about her life. But she used to faint all the time and it happened to her like it happened to us. I didn't know if it was because of the vaccine because she was in a different class, because of the separation of different classes we didn't talk but she did faint. And now, thinking back, I recall saying to my mother, "Mom, do you remember that I used to tell you about a girl who fainted? Don't you think it was because of the vaccine?"

And she told me, "Maybe, Rosa," because by that time they were vaccinating. But she left and I don't know anything further about her life.

How was your life before the vaccine?

My life before the vaccine was, well... I always was and I am a studious person; that is what I think about myself. I finish everything that I start. I like to be studying, to be researching, to be investigating, to be here and there, to express my opinions. Before the vaccine I talked a lot, expressed my opinions, but afterwards I felt afraid to talk. But thanks to a teacher who was always inquiring, though I felt my heart pounding when she was asking, I told myself that though I felt that I couldn't, I had to respond to her. I was afraid that I would be talking and then all of a sudden I'd fall down and faint; do you understand me?

But I have had to learn to live with this. A doctor told me, "You have to learn how to live with this, the same way that people live with cancer, you have to learn to live with this."

Okay, yes, I have to learn to live with an illness. But people who have cancer have a treatment, they have hope; but we don't know if this is going to go away in one or two years, if this is going to affect us all our lives, or if we are going to be able to have children.

There are many classmates and friends that I have, thanks to the vaccine I have made friends who are in this same situation, and because they have something wrong with their ovaries, they have cysts on their ovaries, they won't be able to have children. They are taking that away from us.

They are violating our right to have children, our rights, the women and the girls of this area are being deprived of the right to have a family.

When my mother mentions my going to the university, they say, "No, if you faint you are not going to study." It is as if they are taking away our right to obtain an education. The fact that we are sick, that we may faint, that we may feel ill with a headache, doesn't mean that we cannot move ahead in life.

But we also need treatment, we need something constant, we need hope, we need to be told, "With this, your illness will go away."

We have been victims of swindlers who promise us cures, who come and say: "This will be good for your daughter." And what they sell is just a boiled herb inside a jar. That is all, and that doesn't work.

Have the doctors from here or from Cartagena told you what your illness is?

No. They say... I used to feel a lot of pain in my chest that pain is not so recurrent, but the headache is. A doctor told me: "Your cardiac rhythms are a little crazy."

That was the diagnosis that I got. They performed a CAT scan on me and it didn't show anything. Everything was normal. The mysterious thing is that everything comes out normal.

When my sister went to the hospital, the nurse used to say about her, "She is one of the normal ones," because everything came out normal. My sister, with her legs crooked, and everything came out normal?

At any point, were you tested for heavy metals?

Heavy metals...

Lead or aluminum in your blood?

Yes, I was tested when we had had blood tests at the hospital, but everything was normal...

Did you receive the results?

The strange thing was that I was taken to a man who performed a test for heavy metals. He put a little tube in my hand and told me, "You have this; this metal is high, your mercury is at this level, this is high, this is low."

But at the hospital the results don't show anything. Whom am I to believe?

How do you think your quality of life could improve if you were recognized as having side effects of the vaccine here in Carmen?

First of all, I'm happy the way I am, with my family; as you can see we are a humble family. We don't have any luxuries... What I want is treatment, I don't expect to receive money. I want to receive treatment and to get help to study, to go ahead with my life, because with this many doors are closed to women, to the young women who are suffering from this. I want a course of treatment so I can say, "Wow, it helped me, I feel healthy, I feel good, I feel I have more strength." Then, they could give me the opportunity to continue studying.

Have the doctors ever told you that your illness was caused by the vaccine?

No.

They don't want to see that?

The illogical part is that when we go to the hospital, I have said that I'm a girl who was vaccinated.

"Don't say that, that you are vaccinated. You have psychological problems." they say. "You are in bad psychological shape because everything is in your mind."

Fine, everything is in my mind because one's disposition is created by the mind. But, how could I want to faint, make a fool of myself in front of a lot of people, because this not only happens at home? When I or the other affected girls are just walking, we all feel the same pain, we all feel the dizziness and we all fall down. We are sent to the psychologist. I told her that I have a disease caused by the vaccine.

She said, "You are not sick," literally scolding me.

Okay, we are ill, but even if you want to say that we are not truly ill, just a little sick, don't scold us, offer us guidance instead. Psychologists are supposed to help us, not to scold us, saying "You are not ill, it isn't the vaccine."

They defend the vaccine chicanery, that it isn't because of the vaccine, that the vaccine is fine. The vaccine was supposed to do some good for us, but they knew of certain effects the vaccine could cause in our bodies. Why didn't they tell us? Then, once informed, it would have been our decision if we wanted the vaccine or not.

There wasn't any informed consent and you were never told about the adverse effects…?

No. I was a minor when that happened. They didn't say, "We are going to have a meeting with the parents to inform them that the girls are going to be vaccinated."

They said that this didn't happen because of the vaccine, but at the school where I was studying in Caracolí, they vaccinated, and the majority of the girls, almost all of them, fainted. By that time of the year, it was raining and they couldn't reach one school, I think it was San Carlos, and the girls from that school have never fainted, they don't suffer from headaches, nothing, and they weren't vaccinated. They weren't able to vaccinate there.

Where is San Carlos located?

Is in a subdivision of Caracolí to the left, it is about 15 minutes from here, by car. I don't think they were vaccinated and they have never suffered from fainting, nothing.

If this was caused by collective stress, fathers, mothers, older people, the teachers, everyone would be fainting, everybody would have a headache; everybody would be suffering and crying with the pains, because they are very strong pains. I used to have chest pain, abdominal pain, pain in my hands, my hands used to get twisted, my sister's face got twisted, like a person who has had thrombosis, facial paralysis, paralysis of the legs… There is a series of complications and effects that this has caused, but we haven't been told that we have this or that, we have no diagnosis.

When was the last time that you fainted?

When was the last time that I fainted? In November, I don't remember the exact date, but I know that it was a Saturday. I study on Saturday and I arrived here from the university, I was getting off the motorcycle. I said, "Mom, where are you?" I couldn't find her. I had a lot of pain in my chest and dizziness and I fell.

When my mother arrived, she saw me lying on the ground. The pain starts and I feel like I'm being asphyxiated and I feel my neck swelling. It is horrible not to be able to breathe, it's horrible.

I don't feel that any young woman is going to make that up, what for? What is the purpose for me to make up that I'm fainting? There are doctors who say, "You're making that up," and the nurse adds, "You need a man." They have fought with us, with the ones who are sick. They throw us on a stretcher and we have to wait for an hour-and-a-half for them to give us IV fluids.

The attention is very inhumane. In this world we are supposed to go to the hospital for them to treat us, because we are not feeling well, because we are sick; for them it is as if a dog had arrived.

You said something important, that you feel that they have taken away from you the opportunity to be mothers and to have relationships. How has it been to relate to other people, to classmates at the university who may not be familiar with your case? How is it to fall in love in your condition? How do you feel about being with somebody or in case you want to have children?

Thank God that in my field of study all of my classmates are females. I told them that I was one of the vaccinated girls; that I faint, that I might be well right now but tomorrow who knows if I will be fine, that I may be fine right now, but who knows if I will be fine in two minutes.

If I say that I have a headache, they say, "Darling, take a pill." We share an understanding.

And in the area of romance, people already know about us, the man knows what I have, if he really loves me, he accepts me. I haven't had any problem with this issue.

Thank God my classmates are very understanding, I tell them what I feel and they are there for me. Thank God I have never fainted there, but a classmate did faint there, and all my classmates acted like nurses, they picked her up and took her to the infirmary, they carried her themselves. There is a lot of unity, it is very humanitarian on their part; they don't want me to see my classmate suffering, and ask me to relax and offer me water. "Don't look over there" they tell me, because people sometimes say, "She got affected and fainted." That could happen because where I used to study most of my classmates saw that a girl fainted and that she started to have seizures and they got so affected that some might have fainted too, but I was never like that. I helped my sister, I talked to her, I gave her massages, I never fainted because I was nervous.

Do you feel it is necessary to tell people what is going on with you to be able to relate to people, and in case something happens to you... do you tell them?

Yes, with my classmates I do, I have told them and since this is something that everybody knows, now it is something very natural that any young woman says, "I have crises." It is like an everyday event. You can look healthy, strong, in good shape, you can get dressed and go to a party. But then, you have to leave it because you are afraid of fainting.

"What are you feeling? What is wrong? You look yellow." Some people criticize me without knowing what my condition is, "You look yellow; you have a strange look on your face." I respond that I have crises that I suffer from this. Although I don't like that word 'suffer' because in reality sometimes God gives you a test that you can endure.

God doesn't give you a weight that you can't carry. That is my opinion and I pray to God every day to help me, so I am able to go ahead with my life, to help me to overcome this and that over time this will leave our bodies.

This is not a mental problem. Those are lies the doctors tell, they say the doctors know. I can't say for sure that they don't know, they may know what they do, but they are not inside our thoughts to say, "Look, you are thinking that you are going to faint, and then you faint."

It is not like that. I don't think that any young woman would want to faint...

Your attitude and strength are very important, like your good judgment and the way you analyze things. There are many girls like you with these issues but who don't have a positive attitude, what would you say to those girls?

I would tell them to trust in God, it is the only thing. To trust in God and to trust their abilities to go ahead with their lives. A positive attitude acts like a treatment.

Actually, my mother is very understanding, the same with my stepfather. They say that stepfathers are bad, but not mine. He is very understanding. And I think that having positive thinking makes you stronger. The solution is not to cut my veins or to take a rope and hang myself.

God gives every person a load and it is just the load that He knows that we are able to carry. I have gone through many very difficult situations. I have been the butt of the jokes, especially from my male classmates when I was studying. They would mock me for having a crisis and it was a very embarrassing situation.

But, I would say, "I don't want to be like this by my own will. This is something that I can't control."

I put all my trust in God once when I had very bad crisis and in a moment when I was able to breathe I said, "Mom, I don't want to be like this; God, please cure me." And after that, I prayed for a half an hour to God, "God, help me, I'm not a bad girl, cure me." And thank God, I improved a real lot. I wasn't fainting every day, after that I had three crises, but they were mild ones, I only had the pain in the chest... Everything depends on the faith one has, on one's positive attitude, and on keeping busy. My message is to have faith in God, and to trust in your own capabilities.

What would you say to city girls who were going to use this vaccine?

I would tell them, from my personal point of view, don't get vaccinated. The vaccine may be legal, but we are talking about your health, think before you act. It's true that cervical cancer has killed many women, but remember that this is very painful, the crises, the fact that you have to be in a hospital for hours, and the fainting, the fact that you cannot fulfill your dreams the way you would want to.

For example, I want to go to Cartagena, to study there, to become a professional there, but I can't. And due to my current condition, I don't know if I'm going to faint or if I'm going to have a headache, or if I might fall and suffer a fracture.

If I'm in a classroom, for example in my profession of being a schoolteacher of small children, and I faint, who is going to help me there if I'm dealing with small children? It is important to think about this, to think about the future...

I'm not saying that all vaccines are bad, but many questions have arisen here... They say that the vaccine was expired, that it was warm... I don't know if the ones they have legalized are good or bad or worse than the ones they used with us.

I do believe that they should research, they should think before they are vaccinated, despite the fact that the government says that this wasn't caused by the vaccine because it is inconvenient for them to say otherwise.

I would tell them to think about it and look at the example of the girls who really have suffered; they have suffered a lot, from one thing and another. To look and learn by walking in someone else's shoes. It is said that you learn from your own experiences, but one also has to learn from and to analyze the experiences other girls have had.

I'm not the only one, there are thousands of girls like me. If they don't want to go through the situation that we are going through, they shouldn't get vaccinated, it is as easy as that.

Epilogue

This book has taken you on a journey to more than a dozen countries spanning the globe. You have visited countries where HPV vaccinations are recommended, mandated, or offered on a 'trial' basis. You have visited every continent on the planet.

You read about families whose previously healthy children experienced new medical conditions, including death, shortly after HPV vaccine administration. You shared their quest for successful treatment protocols. You have been invited to 'walk a mile' in their shoes.

You traveled with families who were told their child's new symptoms were coincidental, manifestations of mass hysteria, invented by their parents, typical 'teen' problems, or psychological in origin only to be vindicated years later with a valid medical diagnosis. Those who received a medical diagnosis had parents who would not give up trying to find a way to restore their child's health at any cost.

You have taken journeys with parents who lost their child after HPV vaccinations. You shared their grief. You shared their anguish when coroners could not determine a cause of death. You shared their quest to find answers from medical/scientific professionals around the world, often at their own personal expense. Some of them were successful; others were not. Some could not afford to continue the search and had to simply accept 'undetermined cause of death' as an answer for the loss of their child. You have witnessed the aftermath of every parent's worst nightmare.

You met families who feel betrayed by the medical system they trusted.

You did NOT meet any families who were anti-vaccine. They would not be facing the issues they are now forced to deal with if they had not believed in vaccines.

What did these parents hope to gain by sharing their stories?

- They hoped to help everyone understand they are not statistics; they are real people trying to deal with issues they never dreamed possible.
- They hoped to help people recognize the possibility that new medical conditions might be associated with HPV vaccine administration.
- They hoped to inspire medical professionals to work with each other across multiple disciplines to find successful treatment protocols.
- They hoped to convince medical professionals the same informed choice mandatory with any other health intervention, must be provided before HPV vaccine administration.
- They hoped to inspire scientists to conduct studies to determine who is most susceptible to adverse reactions after HPV vaccines and why, so these people can be protected in the future.
- They hoped government representatives and health officials would recognize the possibility that their children's new medical conditions might be HPV vaccine-related.
- They hoped to convince government health officials to include the potential risks of HPV vaccines as well as promised, yet to be proven, benefits when determining the risk/benefit profile of this medical intervention.
- They hoped to convince legislators and health officials to stop trying to mandate medical procedures.
- They hoped to make sure everyone knows how important it is for healthcare decisions to be left in the hands of parents and their medical professionals.

Are any of these hopes unreasonable?

- Is it ethical to administer a medical intervention without providing the prospective recipient with enough information to make an informed choice?
- Is it ethical to risk a person's health and well-being, perhaps their life, on the 'altar of the greater good'?

- Is it ethical to ignore potential unintended consequences when they do occur?
- Is it ethical to treat people as if they are psychotic, hysterical, or simply unimportant when they report unusual symptoms after medical procedures?
- Is it ethical for politicians and administrative health officials to make medical decisions for you and your family?
- Do politicians and administrative health officials know more about your family history than you and your medical provider?

Most of these questions boil down to asking whether or not every single human life matters. If every life matters, then some substantial changes to current medical paradigms need to be made.

Will you stand by until you make your own journey from trust to tragedy, or will you stand beside families who made the journey before you?

The choice is yours.

Remember, individually we can help; together, we can make a lasting difference.